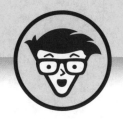

Foam Rolling

by Mike D. Ryan, PT, ATC

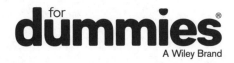

for dummies®
A Wiley Brand

Foam Rolling For Dummies®

Published by: **John Wiley & Sons, Inc.**, 111 River Street, Hoboken, NJ 07030-5774, www.wiley.com

Copyright © 2021 by John Wiley & Sons, Inc., Hoboken, New Jersey

Published simultaneously in Canada

For general information on our other products and services, please contact our Customer Care Department within the U.S. at 877-762-2974, outside the U.S. at 317-572-3993, or fax 317-572-4002. For technical support, please visit https://hub.wiley.com/community/support/dummies.

Wiley publishes in a variety of print and electronic formats and by print-on-demand. Some material included with standard print versions of this book may not be included in e-books or in print-on-demand. If this book refers to media such as a CD or DVD that is not included in the version you purchased, you may download this material at http://booksupport.wiley.com. For more information about Wiley products, visit www.wiley.com.

Library of Congress Control Number: 2020949681

ISBN 978-1-119-75732-0 (pbk); ISBN 978-1-119-75733-7 (ebk); ISBN 978-1-119-75734-4 (ebk)

Manufactured in the United States of America

SKY10022968_120220

Contents at a Glance

Table of Contents

Introduction

"A journey of a thousand miles begins with a single step" is a famous Chinese proverb attributed to Lao Tzu. As a sports medicine specialist, physical therapist, former National Football League Head Athletic Trainer and six-time Ironman triathlete, I playfully remind my patients, "A journey of a thousand miles begins with a single *roll*."

I want to congratulate you on taking your first step to gaining control of your body by seeking the skills to master the use of rollers. I see way too many people with chronically tight muscles and painful joints seeking complex and expensive means to restore their muscle and joint mobility. Too often, they overlook simpler and inexpensive solutions, like rollers and roller balls, as a trusted tool to reduce their muscle pain without medicine.

Humbled by the impact of the COVID-19 pandemic, most of us, myself included, have come to the realization that our most treasured human possession is our health. My passion as a sports medicine specialist is to help people just like you to manage your pain using safe and effective techniques without medicine. That is why I've focused a large part of my physical therapy treatments to include rollers, half rollers, roller balls, and vibrating rollers.

About This Book

This book is for you. I'll share with you sports medicine tips normally reserved for elite, professional athletes. This book will help you master roller treatments, workouts, and stretches to reduce your muscle pain and increase your joint mobility.

Rollers will change your life. You'll learn to scout your body for painful muscle restrictions, quickly unlock tight muscles, perform targeted strengthening exercises, and finish with tailored functional drills to keep you pain-free.

We'll start with everything you need to know about the rollers themselves — the round ones, the ball ones, the half ones, and even the vibrating ones. Next, you'll look at all the muscles and stuff under the skin that you'll be treating with those rollers. Becoming familiar with tight muscles, bound-down fascia, trigger points, and scar tissue will make you an expert at fixing your nagging aches and pains quickly just like world-class athletes do.

The next five chapters is the "fun part," says the physical therapist. You'll learn 56 muscle-unlocking treatments, neatly arranged into five treatment zones:

>> Upper leg

>> Lower leg and foot

>> Lower back and hips

>> Chest, upper back, lats, and neck

>> Shoulders and arms

After your muscles are unlocked, loose, and limber, they're perfectly primed for the challenging roller workouts found in Chapter 21. Your key muscles will be targeted for both strengthening and lengthening with your new versatile training partner: your roller.

We all have aches and pains that try to slow us down. They won't succeed if you implement the pain-eliminating game plans found in the injury management chapter, Chapter 22. I'll share with you my easy-to-follow sports medicine checklist developed to safely return injured professional athletes back on the field.

Lastly, this book provides another level of support for your health and wellness by helping you to stay injury-free by customizing your injury prevention game plan. All you need to do is plug in your sport, and you'll be given customized treatments, strengthening drills, and preventative exercises to keep you injury-free.

Foolish Assumptions

I didn't write this book solely for professional football players or Ironman triathletes, who I've treated for a majority of my professional career. As I wrote this book, I made some assumptions about you, the reader.

I assume you're a hard-working, non-professional "athlete," who wants to stay very active and healthy as you juggle a full-time job, a significant other, children, a moderately active social life, and, a few nagging injuries that just don't seem to go away.

You have a roller or two but you don't use them too often. And when you do, you just kind of roll them around "here and there on the sore spots" in an effort to warm up your muscles. You hear others talk about rolling, but you don't "get" it based on your limited use of the rollers.

My assumptions continue:

>> You dream of moving pain-free without stiffness or limitations throughout your busy day.

>> You strongly yearn to be active, youthful, and happy.

>> Sweating is a form of cleansing for your body, mind, and soul.

>> You're scared of your body get old too soon with so many cool things waiting for you on your Bucket List.

>> You're tired of being in pain.

>> You're starting to make funny noises when you get out of low chairs or pick up anything off the floor. (Oh, no! You're sounding like an old person!!)

>> You're tired of doctors and medical specialists not taking your complaints and frustrations seriously.

>> You're tired of personal trainers showing you cool workouts that feel fine for a week or two until the pain takes you back to where you started: in pain and out of shape!

>> You're tired of your old body not keeping up with your youthful mind.

>> You're willing to put in the work to get rid of your pain if someone credible gave you simple, proven directions on what you need to do.

>> And *when* you are healthy, you're more than willing to do your daily maintenance work to stay pain-free!

Icons Used in This Book

Throughout the book, I use a handful of icons to point out various types of information. Here's what they are and what they mean:

REMEMBER

The Remember icon is like a little sticky note, labeling everything in the book that's key to remember.

TIP

The Tip icon indicates a quick way to remember important material or perform a task. Use these tips to help you improve your health and wellness.

WARNING

The Warning icon helps you steer around mistakes that active people commonly make. Don't let them happen to you!

OUCH

The Ouch icon highlights material related to pain. It helps you recognize when an injury or treatment might be uncomfortable so that you can keep your eye on the prize: *pain-free movement.*

PT NOTE

The Physical Therapy Note reminds you when the author is putting on his physical therapy hat to share sports medicine tips to help you master the art of self-myofascial muscle unlocking with rollers, roller balls, and handheld massagers.

Beyond the Book

As if there isn't already a ton of great information in this book, you can also access the book's Cheat Sheet at dummies.com. This Cheat Sheet provides quick and handy info and tips you can use on the go. It includes a body assessment, easy and hard roller workouts injury prevention with rollers and more.

To access this Cheat Sheet, simply go to www.dummies.com and search for "Foam Rolling For Dummies Cheat Sheet."

Where to Go from Here

The layout of this book makes it easy for you to learn everything you need to know to become a master roller. You can read it from front to back or jump into a chapter to address your immediate needs. The simple titles of both the parts of the book and the chapters make it easy for you to find what you're looking for quickly.

Chapter 1 is a great introduction to the wonderful world of rolling. It will help answer many of the questions novice rollers commonly have. After that, continue onto Chapter 2 or consult the Table of Contents and jump in anywhere you like. I use plenty of cross-references so you know where to go if you need more information about a particular topic.

1
Getting Started with Rolling

Chapter **1**

Rolling for Life

Welcome to the first physical therapy–based roller treatment book with easy-to-follow treatment programs. After using the treatments and workouts in this book, you'll never look at your rollers in the same way again.

I'm assuming that you purchased *Foam Rolling For Dummies* for one of three reasons:

>> You have a roller, but you don't really know how to use it properly.

>> You're looking for an effective way to keep you body moving like it did ten years ago.

>> You're tired of being in pain or always being injured.

If so, you're reading the perfect book for you. All three are great reasons to learn how to use a muscle roller in the right way.

TIP

I want to clarify a terminology issue before we start our journey together. The title of this book obviously includes "Foam Rolling." While you will be using some foam rollers with your muscle treatments, I'll refer to all of them simply as "rollers." Many of the rollers, roller balls, vibrating rollers, and roller sticks I use are made of a variety of materials other than foam.

The Mind of an All-Pro Roller

I worked for 26 years in the National Football League (NFL) in a hands-on role as the Head Athletic Trainer/Physical Therapist. I learned the art of teaching sports medicine techniques to elite athletes to help them both manage their injuries and optimize their ability to move pain-free. I want to share those same sports medicine skills, normally reserved for world-class athletes, with you and your roller.

This game plan starts with teaching you to think about using rollers in your daily routine. Knowing when and when not to use a roller or roller ball is extremely important in order to stay safe. Understanding the following benefits of rollers will help you effectively apply them to your busy schedule each day:

>> They improve posture after a great night of sleep.

>> They loosen tight muscles before exercise.

>> They reduce pain in a trigger point or a "knot" in a muscle.

>> They accelerate recovery following exercise.

REMEMBER

This is not your typical how-to book. I'm not taking the easy route by simply telling you to "use this roller for that injury" or "roll like this." You've spent your hard-earned money to purchase this book, and you deserve better.

Understanding the many amazing uses of a roller will help you apply the roller treatments in Chapters 16 to 20. Each treatment in the five body zones and the challenging roller workouts has a progression structure built in to help you accelerate your improvements. I'll help you think like an *all-pro roller*, knowing exactly when to ramp your roller treatments and workouts up or down.

Rollers 101

Finding the right roller for you is the smart place to start. With so many variables when it comes to rollers, this task is not as easy as it sounds. Rollers vary in shape, size, material, uses, and mechanical vibrations. Because of the wide range of roller traits, they provide a wide range of benefits.

To help select the perfect roller for you, let's assume you're experiencing muscle tightness. You desperately want to run in the local 5K road race this weekend, so you need to reduce the muscle tightness and its associated pain.

With this scenario in mind, here are a few examples to help you select the best roller for you:

>> **Pain is located in the front (quadriceps), back (hamstrings), outside (iliotibial band), or inside (groin) of the thigh.**

 Use a cylindrical full roller (see Chapter 2).

>> **Pain is located in the lower, outside corner of the shin.**

 Use a round, hard roller ball (see Chapter 17).

>> **Pain is located in the lower back and outside corner of the hip.**

 Use a half roller (see Chapter 18).

After selecting the perfect roller for you, you need to find a safe place to roll. I don't want you getting injured while rolling, so your "launch pad" to roll needs to be risk-free. Rolling surfaces can include a carpeted floor, a hard wall, backyard grass, dirt in a campground, or a wooden gym floor. The key safety tip is to have plenty of space, with no risky obstacles nearby disguised as pets, sharp objects, children, unstable objects, or sporting equipment.

Getting Under Your Skin

If you're like most people, you're looking for safe and effective ways to stay healthy. This starts with understanding what's really going on under your skin. If you think the same, well, I have you covered in Chapters 10 to 15. It won't earn you a medical degree, but you'll love my "keep it simple" teaching style helping you to understand your body's inner workings. Together, we'll walk through cool topics like muscles, fascia, trigger points, pain, scar tissue, nerves, and posture.

As an example, when your muscles are forced to work hard in a limited range of motion, they become tight and restricted. Think of the last time you had to carry a heavy bag in your hand for a prolonged period of time. Maybe you were carrying heavy luggage through the airport or groceries in from the car. Regardless, your finger flexor muscles quickly became tight and painful.

This would be a simple example of tight, overworked muscles and fascia that would benefit from a two- to three-minute rolling treatment from Chapter 20 using a roller ball.

Tight fascia wrapped around all your muscles, bones, organs, and joints will limit your mobility. Roller treatments are quick solutions to keep your fascia and muscles loose and limber. Unlike long flexibility classes and tedious flexibility routines, the roller treatments found in Chapters 16 to 20 focus on the source of the tightness — painful trigger points — which can be eliminated in less than five minutes!

Key Questions for You

The power of this book lies in both your hands and your mind. This book gives you the ability to take ownership of your muscles and how they function. Too often, I see individuals blindly hand their health and livelihood over to someone else. In doing so, a vast majority of the responsibility for that patient's health, activity level, and attitude is guided by their doctor, family members, spouse, physical therapist, personal trainer, and so on. That type of passive approach is a formula for a sub-par outcome.

Instead, I encourage my patients to take an active approach to their health. I don't recommend that you "go rogue" and blaze your own trail back to a healthy you. But I do encourage you to build your own wellness team with skilled and caring specialists while keeping yourself firming positioned in the driver's seat.

To find the right answers as the captain of your wellness team, you must start with some key questions.

How do I unlock my thigh and hamstrings muscles?

Prolonged sitting, walking in dress shoes, and standing on hard surfaces typically results in tight and painful quads and hamstrings. These restricted muscles struggle to flush out waste products as they desperately scream for the inflow of fresh, oxygen-heavy, healthy blood.

Besides your audible grunts and groans, your simple active movement can become labored and strenuous. After periods of prolonged sitting or standing, do your legs feel like you're wearing a pair of jeans that are two sizes too small? If so, then you'll love Chapter 16. You'll learn how to unlock your thigh muscles, as shown in Figure 1-1, to regain pain-free muscle mobility and flexibility.

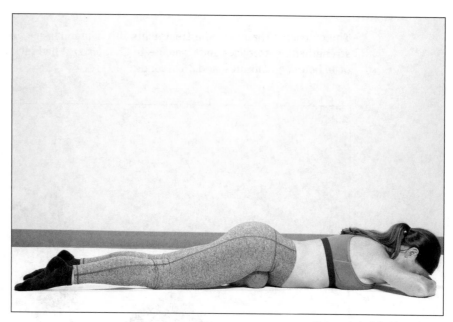

Photography by Haim Ariav & Klara Cu

FIGURE 1-1: Unlocking the hard-working upper quadriceps muscles.

Why do my lower legs always seem to be my troublemaking "Achilles heels"?

Your quads may get all the hype in the beach photos, but your shin muscles have certainly earned the need for some love. Your calf muscles on the back, peroneal muscles on the outside, and ankle dorsi flexor muscles on the front of the shins are the unsung heroes of your active lifestyle.

Your shins and their many muscles, tendons, fascia, and ligaments have a difficult task of keeping you balanced while battling with the ground on each and every step. Because of this, when any of the muscles in your shin or foot become tight or injured, the results can be painful.

Training for my sixth Ironman triathlon in Austria at the age of 46, I strained my calf three times! The last muscle injury, five weeks before my big race, was so severe that I had to break off small branches of a tree to build a mock heel lift for my shoes just to be able to limp home.

The outcome: Thanks to the treatments in Chapter 17 (see Figure 1-2) and the strengthening exercises and stretches in Chapter 21, I had my personal best time of 10 hours, 36 minutes, and 46 seconds.

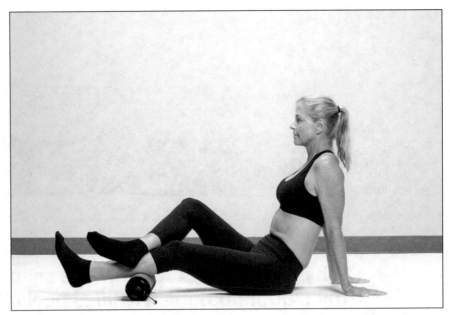

Photography by Haim Ariav & Klara Cu

FIGURE 1-2:
Roller
treatment
for a tight calf.

If I could make my lower back and hips pain-free, would it make my life easier and more fun?

If this question made you smile and nod with approval, hurry on to Chapter 18 to make your *happy lower back* dream a reality. I say that because lower back pain is so common in today's society. Chances are good that you experience painful lower back symptoms on a daily basis. This is a sad fact that I want to significantly reduce with this book.

If you've experienced lower back or hip pain, you'll recognize some of the symptoms noted in Figure 1-3, represented by the "roof" and the "ladder." The roof represents your three gluteus muscles, while the ladder represents your hip external rotator muscles entwined with your sciatic nerve.

If you suffer from pain in either of those two regions, the secret roller ball treatment plans in Chapter 18 will change your life! The step-by-step protocol to unlock painful lower back and hip muscles is the same treatment used by professional football players preparing for their NFL games.

How can I improve my posture to relax my chest, upper back, and neck?

It's kind of a chicken-and-egg type of a dilemma. What comes first: tightness at the base of your neck or in your chest muscle? Either way, your shoulders become rounded, your chin protrudes forward, and your neck becomes tight and sore. With prolonged sitting and working at the computer, both your symptoms and posture will worsen.

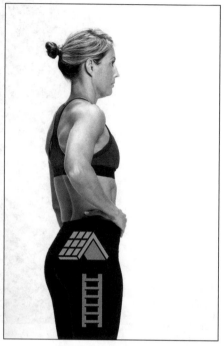

Photography by Haim Ariav & Klara Cu

FIGURE 1-3:
Unlock glute muscles on the "roof," and hip external rotators on the "ladder."

Look around. You're not alone. The proven sports medicine tricks that you need are in this book, as shown in Figure 1-4. Those posture-improving tricks can be found in Chapter 19.

How can I eliminate my shoulder and arm pain with a small roller ball?

If you suddenly got excited and snapped into a daydream about playing tennis again, well, Chapter 20 was written just for you!

After 26 years of working with professional football players, I want to share with you the tricks used to unlocking their strong, and often painful, shoulders. The easy-to-follow technique, shown in Figure 1-5, wisely uses the stronger shoulder muscles to unlock the weaker, tighter muscles with the help of a roller ball.

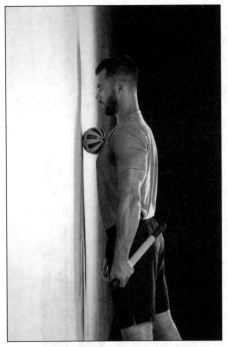

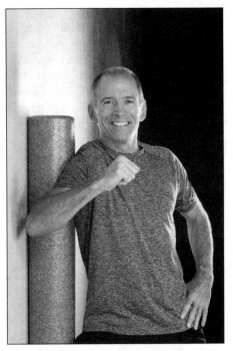

Photography by Haim Ariav & Klara Cu

Photography by Haim Ariav and Klara Cu

FIGURE 1-4:
Unlocking the pectoralis minor allows the entire shoulder girdle to naturally glide backwards.

FIGURE 1-5:
Unlocking the shoulder external rotator muscles inside "the scapular triangle."

Chapter 20 is packed with fast-acting roller treatments for your shoulders and arms.

Working Out with Rollers

Roller treatments are perfect for reducing your pain, relaxing your muscles, and getting you back into "your game." Your game may be tennis, running, swimming, hiking, yoga, biking, or anything that makes you happy and enhances your health. Now you're ready to take your game to a new level with the help of your versatile roller.

Roller workouts help you improve your body in four ways:

» Muscle strength

» Muscle endurance

>> Muscle and fascia length

>> Body balance

Take a moment to review those four important body benefits. Now envision how much your body and lifestyle would improve if each of those four traits improved by a mere 20 percent!

OUCH

The workouts and stretching section in Chapter 21 will challenge you to the max! I was forced to do my obstacle course training workouts at home during the 2020 COVID-19 pandemic quarantine. I developed a series of two-level roller workouts for the upper body, core, and lower body, which I'm very proud of. If you feel like laughing and scoffing at "lame workouts on rollers," you just might want to put those workouts to the test before you laugh at them in public. Trust me, they're much harder than you think.

Using Rollers to Manage Your Injuries

PT NOTE

We all seem to have our share of aches and pains. Certain activities, movements, and even lack of movement while sitting can bring on painful symptoms. Because I'm a physical therapist and athletic trainer, this is my wheelhouse. I'll walk you through *quick* roller treatments to unlock your muscles, decrease your pain, and increase your joint range of motion.

I take great pride in educating non-professional athletes, just like you, to manage your injuries safely with rollers. What you do with your new looser muscles and limber joints is your priority. I've watched my patients, young and old, change their lives with simple rollers and my proven treatment game plans. Instead of just lying on a roller and rolling around, you'll learn easy-to-follow protocols. Each treatment is fast and effective, and most treatments take a mere two to four minutes to complete!

With so many rollers to choose from — full rollers, half rollers, roller balls, vibrating rollers, roller sticks, and even vibrating roller balls — I'll help you to determine exactly which roller is best suited for your ailment or injury.

When you have muscle pain, it's important to find the source of the pain. When most people think about finding the source of their muscle pain, they revert to the age-old mindset of seeking an expensive doctor for expensive tests.

I have a new option that puts you in control of your care. I don't want you to avoid your doctor or healthcare specialists when dealing with severe medical conditions. However, when muscle tightness and pain is limiting your active life-style, I want to empower you to quickly find the source of your pain *and* start your roller treatment.

TIP

My ROLLER Treatment Planner in Chapter 22 is a game changer when it comes to helping you assess your body, isolate your restriction, determine the exact treatment needed, treat the source of your pain, and follow through with preventative exercises to reduce the risk of the pain returning.

The previous paragraph is worth re-reading because it may seem too good to be true.

Let's walk through a quick example of applying my ROLLER Treatment Planner.

>> **Symptoms:** Lower back/hip pain

>> **Finding:** Tight *left* hip flexors, bilateral weak glute muscles, poor posture

>> **Source of pain:** Overly tight *left* glutes

>> **Treatment plan:**

- Half roller treatment, Level 1 — *left* hip flexors

- Roller ball treatment, Level 2 — bilateral glutes

- Bird dogs, Level 2 — bilateral pelvis/shoulders

- Roller hip flexor stretches — bilateral

>> **Preventative exercises:**

- Roller hamstring stretches

- Roller body squats, Level 2

It's that simple. The ROLLER Treatment Planner in Chapter 22 is easy to use, it provides you with a clear solution and, most importantly, it works!

How will you know the muscle and fascia treatments work? In Chapter 16, I'll show you a simple pre-test/post-test that you can do before and after your roller treatments to show you exactly how much your movement has improved. Without spending hours stretching, twisting, and massaging, your improvements in tightness, pain, joint stiffness, and weakness will be felt in less than five minutes!

Seeing people's faces light up with gratitude when they quickly find themselves moving pain-free after months or years of suffering with muscle pain and tightness. This is another example of why I love my career in sports medicine.

Preventing Injuries with Roller Treatments

PT NOTE

Preventative medicine isn't sexy and it's not commonly bragged about on social media. But injury prevention works. If you follow the same simple sports medicine roller techniques I used with my NFL players, your risk of an injury will be drastically reduced. And if you stay injury-free, as my wife will confirm as it relates to me, you'll be much easier to live with!

PT NOTE

I'd like you to think about the following statement for 30 seconds and see if you agree with it:

If you found a way to decrease your pain while increasing your muscle range of motion, you'd be a happier friend, more loving sibling, healthier neighbor, stronger athlete, more caring parent, more focused worker, and better sleeper.

I hope this statement resonates with you, and you agree with the words wholeheartedly.

Both personally and professionally, this is the impact I believe rollers will have on your life. I've witnessed those types of positive impacts on hundreds of people's lives thanks to rollers and the preventative exercises found in Chapter 23.

How would your life and attitude change if your pain was significantly reduced while your muscle and joint range of motion returned to the mobility you experienced ten years ago?

The three steps — unlocking muscles, strengthening opposing muscles, and preventative exercises — in Chapter 23 are perfectly designed for each sport to keep you injury-free. I made it simple: Find your sport. Implement your three steps. Repeat the three steps twice a week. It's that easy.

Preventing injuries becomes more important as we age. None of us heal like we did when we were in our 20s. Therefore, we all need to make preventing injuries a higher priority. Chapter 23 is loaded with roller tips to keep you out of the doctor's office and in the game.

In summary, I hope you find the roller information in this book to be both body- and life-changing. Rollers will make your muscles, fascia, and joints looser and happier. Start slow, follow the treatment guidelines and photos to improve your form. And always listen to your body. Your body knows what it needs to get better, and we can always be better listeners.

Let's rock and roll!

WHY I'M EXCITED ABOUT THIS BOOK

I wrote this book to help people who suffer with pain and limited motion every day. I'm not going to insult you, or myself, by assuming that I can help everyone who's in pain. But I *can* help a large percentage of people suffering from tight muscles, chronically tight fascia, restricted soft tissue, and painful trigger points. Many times a week, people tell me, "I only wish someone told me how to use rollers months ago," or "If I knew how to use these rollers years ago, it would have saved me a lot money and pain!"

It's powerful feedback like this that motivated me to put my roller treatments, workouts, and sports medicine insight into this book.

I've worked aggressively using rollers with patients at every level of fitness and sports. My patients range from professional football players, to weekend warriors, professional golfers, elite high school athletes, Olympians, walking-on-the-beach grandparents, retired NBA basketball players, world-class Ironman triathletes, and everyone in between.

As a six-time Ironman triathlete, former collegiate miler, and extreme sports enthusiast, I use all of the roller techniques and workouts in this book on myself. My routine of rolling two times a day helps me both fine-tune the techniques and better communicate the fine details of each technique to you, the reader.

Chapter **2**

Choosing the Right Roller(s) for You

You're probably reading this book because you roll on a roller now and then to help with your chronic leg pain or a tight hip, with no set roller game plan. Your results are probably encouraging yet not life changing. Meanwhile, you're probably somewhat intrigued by rollers, making you want to find out more. Sure, you see rollers everywhere: at friends' houses, in the gym, on social media, and in online fitness classes. And you may even hear some of your friends bragging about their roller routines.

"Okay, enough already!" you tell yourself. Now both your mind and your chronically sore legs are finally on board to learn how to safely and effectively master the use of a roller.

Next, you do a quick "foam roller" search on Amazon. It stops you in your tracks. You find a whopping seven pages of rollers! Where do you start? There are way too many shapes and sizes to choose from. Suddenly, your head is hurting more than your legs.

Not to worry. In this chapter, I will help you find the perfect roller(s) for you. I explain the differences between rollers and the best uses for each one. Whether you need a roller to relax your shoulder muscles, eliminate painful knots in your thighs, or improve your posture, I will help you adopt the best roller for your needs.

Not All Rollers Are Created Equal

Rollers come in many shapes, sizes, colors, and types of material. And with each of those different types of rollers come many different functions. Just like none of our bodies are the same, not all rollers are created equal. Although the sheer variety of rollers can sometimes be confusing, I'll show you how to optimize your body's benefits from the many roller options available to you.

REMEMBER

The term *foam rollers* is generally used to describe all rollers. Case in point: the title of this book. However, the standard round "foam" roller is just one type of roller you can use to unlock your muscles, increase your joints' range of motion, strengthen your core muscles, and improve your body's health. With that being said, I will consistently refer to these valuable wellness tools as simply "rollers."

Because rollers have such a wide range of uses, no one roller will meet all of your needs. Rollers can be used to treat the spine, shoulders, upper extremities, core, hips, and lower body. Based on the wide range of muscle sizes and body variations, different roller sizes, shapes, and textures can be used throughout the body.

"THIS REALLY WORKS!"

It's not unusual to find even high-level athletes who haven't been exposed to elite sports medicine techniques with rollers. At first, they're skeptical about the benefits of using a roller and the device's role in keeping them healthy.

That's when I love to help them see the results firsthand. These athletes know their bodies better than anyone, me included. Therefore, it's important for them to *feel* the benefits more than for them to simply *hear* the benefits from me or their coach.

I had a young NFL professional football player suffering from chronic hamstring pain who boldly told me, "rollers are a waste of time."

The challenge was on.

I asked the 23-year-old athlete to perform simple walking, marches, and squats to assess how his legs and hips felt. Next, I asked him to select which leg was the tighter of the two. I then walked him through two minutes of rolling that leg. Lastly, I asked him to repeat his exact pre-roll moving routine of walking, marching, and squatting.

The look on his face said it all. I just smiled when he boldly said, "This #@*# (roller) really works!! Man, can I roll my other leg now?"

If you're a beginner, I recommend starting with the basic cylindrical foam roller (shown in Figure 2-1). It's softer, more stable, and more comfortable for introducing someone to proper roller techniques. It may not be as effective for treating smaller, more localized trigger points, but I would rather see you start slower as you learn how to roll and unlock larger muscles on a more comfortable standard roller.

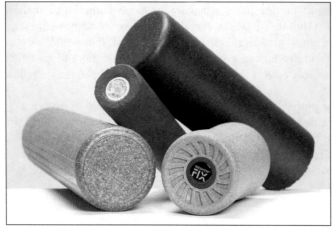

Photography by Haim Ariav & Klara Cu

FIGURE 2-1:
Circular rollers
come in
various sizes
and lengths.

Circular rollers: Keeping it simple

The most basic of rollers is the round cylinder roller, shown in Figure 2-1. Most of them are made of foam. Their diameter is typically 6 inches, while their length can range from 12 inches to 4 feet. Because they are larger and made of a softer material, they will be more comfortable for rookie rollers and those managing more painful ailments.

REMEMBER

Learning all the nuances of rolling will take some time. Learning on a softer and more comfortable roller like a standard circular foam roller will help accelerate or steepen "the learning curve."

OUCH

Some discomfort can be expected when rolling on tight muscles and trigger points. Using softer rollers with a proper technique will help. Harder rollers with a multi-pattern texture isolate the pressure, which can be more uncomfortable. Later in this book you will learn the tricks to minimize the "bad pain" while focusing on the "good pain" of unlocking muscles.

Pro: Softer, more comfortable, larger pressure surface, easy to balance, less expensive.

Con: Less depth of pressure, less localized treatments.

Multi-pattern design rollers

A multi-pattern roller is usually the same diameter, six inches, as the basic foam roller, but its surface is very different. As the name suggests, the rolling surface of a multi-pattern roller is not flat. Instead, these rollers are covered with ridges, pressure pads, and grooves. They often look more like a truck tire than a roller. The inner core of the roller can be foam, hard plastic, or hollow.

The purpose of these rollers, which are shown in Figure 2-2, is to apply more localized pressure on trigger points and scar tissue within skin, muscle, tendons, and fascia while rolling. With its many ridges and angled peaks, a multi-pattern roller allows you to maneuver the peaks of the roller into and around uneven muscles, tendons, and fascia.

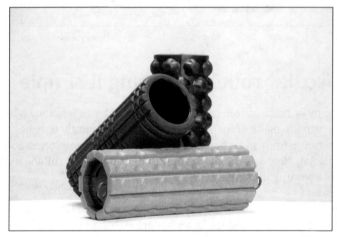

FIGURE 2-2: Multi-pattern rollers provide varying surfaces to treat muscles tendons and fascia tissue.

Photography by Haim Ariav & Klara Cu

OUCH

These rollers are effective at improving tissue mobility yet are more painful during rolling. Unlike the softer foam roller's broad surface, which is applied to a bigger, wider area over a muscle, this varied surface will apply pressure to a smaller, isolated area. Think about the difference between a steak knife and a butter knife. The point of a steak knife has a much smaller contact spot. This makes the knife "sharper" and more painful if applied to your skin.

BOX OF TISSUE TRICK: "LET'S STAY THE COURSE"

Working with professional football players is hard work, rewarding, and entertaining. Their physical and mental toughness is impressive. To motivate them during their injury prevention, rehabilitation, and recovery work, I used their toughness as a way to challenge them.

With rollers and stretching being a big part of their physical therapy maintenance work with me, helping them manage the discomfort of a hard rolling session was a challenge. They appreciated the value of the rollers, but when it came to rolling over dozens of bruises and trigger points the day after a brutally physical NFL game, it was not fun for any of them.

If they complained too much, I used a simple trick to challenge their toughness and to keep them on task: I would smile and quietly put a box of tissues next to them on the floor. It was my way of saying: "If you want to cry, grab a tissue and feel sorry for yourself for a minute, but we will get back to work because we both know this is exactly what you need."

It always worked. It got the message across loud and clear. Many times, the box was thrown back at me, with a few choice words not fit to be put in print! My tissue trick was a simple way of me saying, without words: "Man, I know this hurts, but we both know these rollers are what will get your muscles back to being healthy fast. I'm right here with you, so let's stay the course."

That's when I'd happily grab a roller and join them for a roller treatment as well. I would never ask my athletes to perform a self-myofascial unlocking technique with a roller for which I was not willing to do myself right next to them. Professional credibility with my athletes is extremely important to me.

Pro: Versatile for treatments, more hard-core for heavier body parts.

Con: Not useful for workouts, more painful, moderately more expensive.

Vibrating rollers

"Long Roller and Roller Ball, I'd like to introduce you to Mr. Massage." Here's where high-tech merges with rollers and roller balls. These heavenly tools combine the many benefits of rollers while adding the relaxing effects of a vibrating massage.

These rollers come in many shapes, from the cylindrical shape in Figure 2-3 to the ball shape in Figure 2-4. They have varied degrees of control, such as vibration intensity, programmable waves of vibration, and heat to individualize your rolling experience.

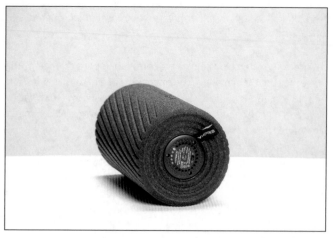

FIGURE 2-3:
Cylindrical
vibrating roller.

Photography by Haim Ariav & Klara Cu

Following are some benefits of vibration therapy:

» Improved circulation

» Decrease in muscle soreness

» Increased soft tissue flexibility

» Improved lymphatic drainage

» Increased tissue temperature

There are many reasons why people benefit from using a roller. Most of those reasons involve soft tissue such as muscles, tendons, fascia, scar tissue, and skin. When you look at that list of tissues being treated, it's easy to see why vibration is beneficial. When any of those soft tissues are relaxed by increasing both the blood flow and the temperature in and between those tissues, they are much easier to treat.

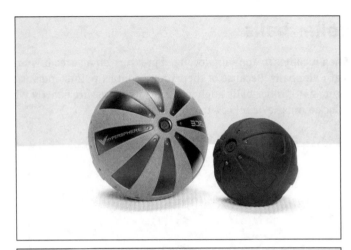

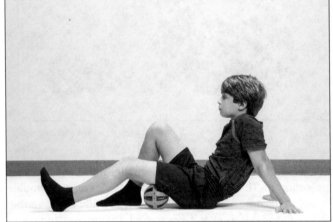

FIGURE 2-4:
Round
vibrating
rollers, large
and small.

Photography by Haim Ariav & Klara Cu

TIP

Tight tissue is typically unhappy tissue. Relaxed, warm, flexible tissue with a rich supply of healthy blood is typically happy tissue.

The cool part about vibrating rollers like the ones shown in Figures 2-3 and 2-4 is that they can also serve as effective rollers without the vibration component turned on. Normal rolling techniques and principles can still be applied if you don't want to use the vibrating element.

Pro: Relaxes body tissue, improved comfort while rolling, versatile for treatments.

Con: More expensive, makes balance more difficult, less useful for workouts.

Roller balls

When it comes to applying localized pressure on an area of your body, it's hard to beat roller balls. Because of their round contact points and varied sizes (shown in Figure 2-5), roller balls apply concentrated pressure exactly where you need it to unlock a muscle or relax a trigger point.

FIGURE 2-5: With their round shape and various sizes, roller balls provide very localized treatments.

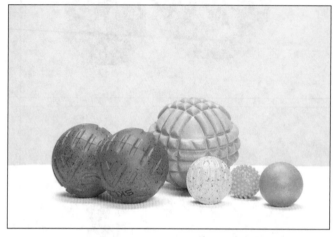

Photography by Haim Ariav & Klara Cu

Roller balls are especially useful for smaller muscles in parts of the body that are more compact. These areas include hands, forearms, shoulders, hips, and feet. You could roll these body parts with a larger roller to warm the area up before you exercise. But if you want to treat those busy areas of the body, a roller ball is the perfect device.

Unlike a typical roller, a roller ball can move in any direction. Where a standard roller functions like a steamroller as it rolls up or down a body part, a roller ball can change direction at any time with a 360-degree range. This hyper mobility is especially helpful when seeking multiple trigger points within a busy area of the body.

Who doesn't love a foot massage?! Here's a special tease: In Chapter 17, I show you how, using the right roller ball and game plan, to give yourself the best foot massage you've ever had!

PT NOTE

It's important to note that more isolated pressure often means a more intense and uncomfortable treatment.

OUCH

Pro: Isolated pressure, more dynamic treatments.

Con: More intense treatments, not useful for workouts.

Half rollers

Half rollers, shown in Figure 2-6, are foam rollers cut in half the long way. The result is a very stable and versatile tool for both treatments and exercise.

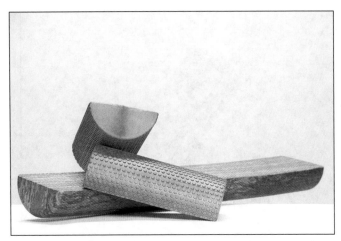

FIGURE 2-6:
Half roller adds
stability to the
standard roller.

Photography by Haim Ariav & Klara Cu

I really like half rollers. For patients who are new to rolling or those who are challenged by balancing on a roller, they are perfect companions. Using half rollers for your shoulders and hips provides a stable roller to relax tight muscles allowing for a deeper treatment. Typically their surface texture is limited, but that does not take away from the many benefits of treating and exercising on a half roller.

PT NOTE

With any of the self-myofascial unlocking techniques for muscles in this book, the half roller is always a safe and simple solution. In other words, if you're doing a treatment on a roller and you're having difficulty maintaining perfect form and relaxing, move to the half roller to improve your technique. This will allow you to breathe normally, maintain perfect positioning on the roller, and unlock your muscles. As you master this technique, you will probably be able to return to a more advanced roller.

Pro: Stable, easier to use, allows longer position holds for postural corrections.

Con: Less dynamic treatments and workouts.

Travel rollers

As the name suggests, travel rollers (Figure 2-7) are collapsible and easy to bring with you on the road. With a simple pull of the strings, the skinny pad is quickly transformed into a stable and functional roller. For years I was forced to be creative when packing my rolling toys when I travelled. I had to pack my underwear, socks, and workout gear inside my roller in my suitcase for my weekly Sunday Night Football game trip. Thankfully, travel rollers have made my packing game plan much easier.

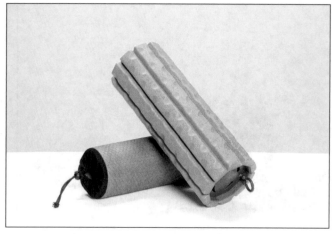

FIGURE 2-7:
Travel roller transforms from a slim travel mate to a solid roller.

Photography by Haim Ariav & Klara Cu

As with the travel roller from Brazyn Life, it offers smooth or multi-patterned surface options. The smoother surface is used like a standard roller with larger contact areas. This allows you to relax larger muscles and larger trigger points. The multi-pattern surface provides multiple contact areas for a deeper treatment.

Pro: Smaller size for travel.

Con: Expensive, fewer size options.

Other Equipment You May Want

Having assistive accessories will help you master the art of rolling. Adding these treatment tools to your body maintenance toolbox will help make your rolling sessions more effective. They will also help you improve your comfort, relaxation, and balance while rolling.

Rolling is not always a simple thing to do. Many factors impact your ability to roll properly. A busy schedule, an uncomfortable injury, attention-hungry kids or pets, and a confined setting are examples of factors that you may have to manage during a roller treatment. The assistive devices listed in the following sections will help improve your roller treatments.

Handheld rollers

Handheld (or *stick*) rollers come in many shapes and sizes. The simple handheld rollers have smoother surfaces (Figure 2-8) or a smaller multi-pattern design (Figure 2-9), like their bigger brothers shown in Figure 2-2.

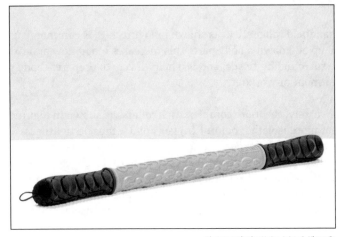

FIGURE 2-8: Simple stick roller for warming up a muscle.

Photography by Haim Ariav & Klara Cu

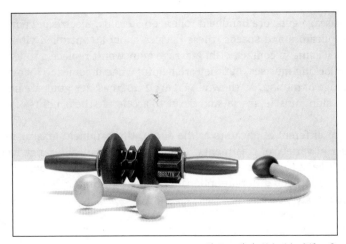

FIGURE 2-9: Complex stick roller to provide isolated muscle treatments.

Photography by Haim Ariav & Klara Cu

They usually have a smaller surface area than a traditional roller, allowing you to localize your treatment area. Because the force applied to the device is mostly controlled manually, you can easily control the amount, direction, and timing of pressure that you apply to treatment areas on your body.

Conversely, when you are lying on a traditional roller, the treatment pressure on the contact area is dependent on four things:

>> Body weight

>> Size and shape of the roller

>> Amount of pressure diverted to the ground by other body parts

>> Good ol' gravity

A handheld roller stick, as shown in Figure 2-8, is commonly used to rhythmically roll up and down a body part. This increases blood flow and tissue temperature in the surrounding tissue, and is a helpful way to prepare a body part for a full roller treatment or workout.

Conversely, the more complex stick rollers, as shown in Figure 2-9, can be used to treat more isolated, painful trigger points, muscle tightness, or scar tissue. I like to think of these types of multi-pattern stick rollers as roller balls with handles. The handles allow for more control in hard-to-reach areas when treating yourself. If someone else is using this type of complex stick roller, it becomes a very useful tool to treat hard-to-reach body parts such as the back corner of the shoulders, the upper hamstrings, and the deep hip muscles.

Handheld massager

Massage guns are handheld rollers on steroids. Electrically powered with various applicators and speeds, these devices apply a controlled vibration to the tissue they come in contact with. Massage guns won't replace a roller when it comes to unlocking muscles, but they are helpful when it comes to increasing healthy joint range of motion. As shown in Figure 2-10, massage guns are helpful for warming up skin, muscle, fascia, and tissue to accelerate the benefits of a roller.

The different applicators at the end of the handheld massagers provide a wonderful variety of treatments. The applicators typically range from medium-size, soft balls to finger-size, hard pointers and anything in between. These applicators allow you different options for applying vibration and massage to any part of your body.

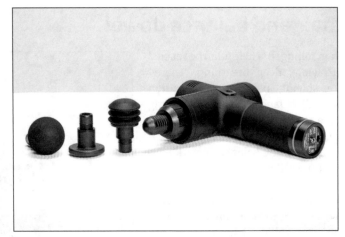

FIGURE 2-10:
Handheld
massager
with varying
speeds and
applicators.

Photography by Haim Ariav & Klara Cu

Let's take a look and see how we would use a handheld massager to prepare for a roller treatment. Say your Achilles tendon is sore. With that you can bet your brain will increase the tension in your calf muscles to protect your Achilles tendon. Those two calf muscles, the gastrocnemius and the soleus muscles, merge together to form your Achilles tendon. This is a perfect opportunity for you to use the handheld massager with the larger, soft ball applicator. It allows you to massage the calf muscles to increase their blood flow, increase the temperature within the muscles, and reduce the tension at the muscle tendons above and below the muscle bellies. This, in turn, allows both muscles to relax, and therefore the stress on your Achilles tendon is reduced. This is an example of the power of sports medicine with roller techniques: significantly reducing your Achilles pain without touching the painful tendon!

Yoga mat

A yoga mat provides an increase in both padding and traction when rolling. It is typically only one-quarter inch thick, so it may not be enough padding if you are rolling over a very hard surface. But using a yoga mat over carpet, padded floor, or firm grass is perfect for rolling.

One of the biggest benefits of using a yoga mat is its traction. Its nonslip surface helps the athlete maintain their position on the roller well, because the yoga mat keeps the roller from slipping.

Chair and balance dowel

When rolling, it's helpful to be relaxed with slow, deep breathing. Therefore, staying in the proper position and well balanced is a must. Using stable objects like a chair, dowel (see Figure 2-11), or wall helps you maintain a stable and balanced position on top of the roller.

Sometimes you will need to be creative in order to maintain proper posture when rolling. I have had to use whatever was available to be able to roll. Not all roller settings are ideal, especially when it comes to rolling while traveling, in the dark, racing, dehydrated, outdoors, on a plane, in excruciating pain, on a boat, or being climbed on by kids or pets.

Following are some of the most unusual items I've used to assist a rolling treatment:

>> Rock

>> Kid

>> Tree

>> Pet dog — my former cat refused to help me. (Hence, "former")

>> Metal soup can

>> Beer bottle

>> Golf ball (Don't try this one at home; it's not for the faint of heart!)

>> Rolled-up magazine

>> Leather belt

>> Trash can

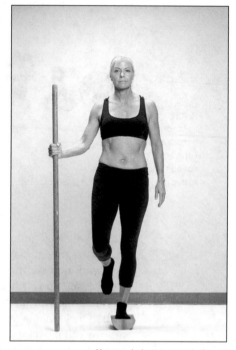

Photography by Haim Ariav & Klara Cu

FIGURE 2-11:
Balance improves with a simple dowel in hand.

Pad and pillows

Being comfortable is important when rolling. Having a properly padded surface or extra pads or pillows (Figures 2-12 and 2-13) is helpful for sensitive, bony body parts such as your elbows, knees, and hips.

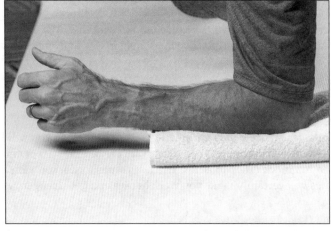

Photography by Haim Ariav & Klara Cu

FIGURE 2-12:
Pad under an elbow equals a happy elbow.

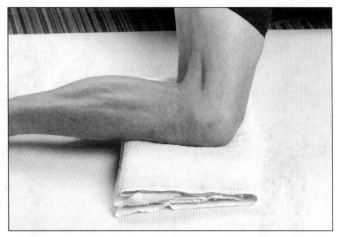

Photography by Haim Ariav & Klara Cu

FIGURE 2-13:
Protecting a bony knee with a pillow or towel.

During some of your rolling treatments, you may feel like a contortionist or a performer for Cirque du Soleil. Having extra padding in areas that may be sensitive will help make you more comfortable.

Stretch bands

Stretch bands are strong bands used to stabilize different parts of your body. They are typically made of rubber or nylon. Stretch bands are used as an extension of your arms, as shown in Figure 2-14, to help move or stabilize your legs, hips, or shoulders. The bands allow you to maintain good posture to protect your spine and joints while rolling for both treatments and workouts.

More advanced treatments include motion with the roller or ball. The bands help to do this when certain joints, like the shoulder, hip, and ankle, are at extreme ranges.

Resistance bands

Resistance bands are, strong rubber bands, as shown in Figure 2-15. Unlike stretch bands, resistance bands are smaller and stretchier. As you will learn in this book, resistance bands can be used to activate certain muscles, while the roller can be used to unlock other muscles. When it comes to workouts on a roller, resistance bands will certainly make you work harder and get stronger faster!

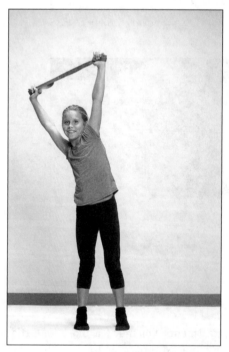

Photography by Haim Ariav & Klara Cu

FIGURE 2-14:
Think of stretch bands as an extension of the arms to properly position a body part.

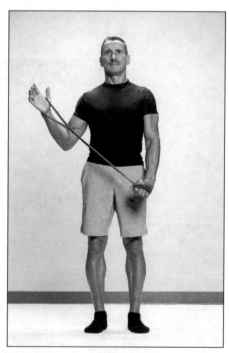

Photography by Haim Ariav & Klara Cu

FIGURE 2-15:
Adding resistance bands helps activate certain muscles while you unlock other muscles.

Finding a Roller to Meet Your Needs

TIP

The deeper you get into the roller world, the more techniques you'll learn to improve your health and active lifestyle. No one roller will meet your needs for treating and exercising all parts of your body.

The following three steps will help you find the perfect roller for your needs:

1. Identify your needs.

Example: "My quads are way too tight."

2. Determine the desired benefit you want from a roller.

Example: "I want my thighs to be more flexible and less painful."

3. Read the corresponding chapter (chapters 16 to 20) related to the body part you plan to treat to find the proper roller and technique to achieve Step 2.

So, for example, if you have tight quads and want your thighs to be more flexible and less painful, head to Chapter 16 to find out what roller is best and what roller treatments to perform to unlock your tight quads.

Chapter **3**
Finding the "Perfect" Roller Launch Pad

I sincerely hope you will find rolling as beneficial for your body and mind as I have. As you learn how to master the art of roller treatments, an important early step is finding a location that helps you roll comfortably in the shortest time possible. I realize that you rarely have the luxury of rolling in a plush fitness studio or on an oceanfront mansion patio. Meanwhile, in the real world, it's important to know what type of setting works best for you.

With many of us now forced to do our workouts outside of public gyms, the places where we do our rolling have also changed. Instead of doing our rolling before our workouts in a spacious gym setting, we now have to be very creative in a new setting. No problem — we got this.

In this chapter, I share easy ways to find or create a safe place to roll. You may not always have a spacious, padded, air-conditioned setting for your roller treatments and workouts. This chapter will show you tips to turn a simple space into your healthy launch pad.

Improvising in Unique Roller Settings

Let's start this search for the perfect roller setting from the neck up. What I mean by this is let's find a way to relax our mind when rolling and then apply that mindset to whatever setting we are in.

TIP

I've learned the value of a relaxed-roller mindset while racing over the last four decades. Those races included six Ironman Triathlons in five countries, muddy Spartan races, mountain obstacle course races, Running of the Bulls in Spain, racing up the Empire State Building in New York City, and New Year's Eve midnight races in Central Park, just to name a few. Each one of those unusual races had unique settings for my pre-race and post-race rolling and stretching sessions.

Extreme races, like the ones I've competed in, are stressful and very challenging. As a result, being properly prepared before each of those races is mandatory to avoid injuries and to perform at a high level. So it would not make sense for me to suddenly not use my rollers the morning of, say, the race up the Empire State Building just because I have to warm up in the lobby of a high-rise building in New York City. Do you think the 86-story-high Empire State Building lobby had a nice, comfortable, padded floor to roll on? No! I was forced to wrap shirts around my elbows and a towel under my knee to be comfortable enough to complete my pre-race rolling routine on the rock-hard tiled floor (#improvise).

When you want to convert some of your space into a roller rink, make it a place you can feel relaxed and safe. Roller rehab and roller workouts should be focused on you. Finding a location where you are safe from injury and your mind can relax is important, especially if you're new to rollers.

Take a moment to look at your home and work settings.

» Is there a solid wall with a clear 4-foot space to use a roller ball in a sock to relax your upper back, as demonstrated in Chapter 19?

» Would your boss even know if you were unlocking your arches (shown in Chapter 17) with a small roller ball under your desk while you typed your weekly reports?

» Your 30-minute-turned-60-minute drive home sure would be less stressful with your roller ball treating the knots in your low back, as shown in Chapter 18, after a hard day at work.

» By simply sliding your living room coffee table to the side, you can turn the carpet between your couch and your TV into the perfect launch pad to roll almost part of your body, as seen in Figure 3-1.

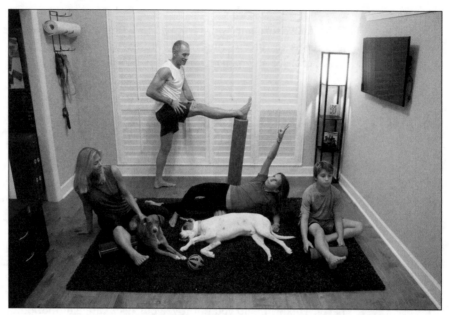

FIGURE 3-1:
Rolling at
home with the
family.

Photography by Haim Ariav & Klara Cu

Finding a Relaxing "Roller Rink"

Each of us has a different definition of a relaxing environment. Some find a dimly lit room to be soothing. Others relax by listening to music. Personally, I find nature sounds and outdoor smells calming.

What type of setting slows your heart rate and gives you a sense of peace? Answering that question is the first step to finding your perfect roller rink. You are probably thinking: "This is starting to sound a lot like meditation." To some degree, you're correct.

TIP

What I mean by this is if you can find a setting that is calm and relaxing for you, it'll lower your heart rate and blood pressure. This, in turn, will help the roller unlock your muscles more quickly so you can perform at a higher level.

How can we turn our "work from home with three kids, two dogs, laundry, dishes, and meals to cook" living room into the perfect roller setting? The answer: by being creative and focusing on having *enough* space rather than the *perfect* space.

Having Enough Room to Roll

Using a roller is a mobile activity, so you'll need some extra real estate. You'll quickly learn how to position yourself in a room or gym to roll properly without ending up bunched in the corner or banging your head on the wall.

You may find yourself having to move furniture to create enough space to roll properly. The good news is that with many of the rolling techniques, you are staying low to the ground. This allows you to slide a leg or arm under a table or bed when rolling in a confined area. Fair warning: when rolling at ground level, you are creating an open invitation for all your pets and children to join your roller party! This will help you improve your neck range of motion, as you will be constantly on the lookout to avoid rolling over little fingers, toes, and tails.

For most lower-extremity treatments and exercises, a 12-x-8-foot carpet or pad is sufficient. When rolling the entire length of the leg or spine, knowing where to start on the pad will help you to still be on the pad when you finish the roll. This is where the "art of rolling" comes into play.

For shoulder, spine, and torso treatments, you also need to have access to a clutter-free and stable wall and doorframe. Doing some of the posterior shoulder and torso treatments with a roller ball on the floor can be painful. With most of your body weight on the ball, the pressure is high and the treatment is intense. By using a wall, the pressure on the trigger point or muscle can be modified. This makes the treatment less intense and more bearable.

A door frame or wall corner is useful when treating the front of the chest and hip. Advanced treatments of these two body parts include active motion along with a roller ball. If these treatments are done against a flat wall, there is a very limited plane of motion because of the wall. But using a door frame or wall corner allows for controlled pressure with the roller ball along with a wide range of active arm or leg motion.

IMPROVISED ROLLER LAUNCH PADS

Few of us can work our lives around our fitness and wellness plans. For most of us, it's the exact opposite: We are forced to work our workouts around our family, jobs, travel, school, and crazy schedule.

I get it. I worked 26 years in the National Football League (NFL) and never took a single sick day. From mid-July to the end of the NFL season, my athletic training staff and I worked seven, yes, 7 days per week. So I get the 'busy, hectic, can't find any free time' schedule thing.

Here are a few "off the beaten path" places I've learned to sneak away to for a quick roller treatment or roller workout:

- **Master bedroom closet:** It's typically carpeted, quiet and spacious. #perfect.
- **Kids' bedroom at night:**
  - *Plan A:* Roll in Gannon's room while he quietly sleeps.

    Plan B: Here's where I shine with my classic Roller Spooky Stories! That's right; you need to master the art of telling great spooky stories to the kids while you roll on their floor. When you do, your kids are super happy, your spouse is thrilled with the free time, and your body is grateful for the unlocking/destressing/relaxation. *That's* a win-win-win!
- **Airports:** Travelling with a roller ball and travel roller turns an airport layover into a physical therapy session. Look for the many tucked-away gates or end-of-terminal spaces to enjoy your favorite music while you unlock your muscles.
- **Parks:** Sitting on a rock-hard bleacher seat watching Makayla play softball is rough on the body, no doubt. Be "that parent" who consistently stretches using the fence or rolls out in the grass behind the left field fence. Instead of worrying about what the other parents might think, soon you'll have them joining you for some "me time" sessions each week.
- **Office break room:** All you need is a roller ball and a longer sock or nylons to turn your office break room wall into a quick de-stressor zone. In less than 10 minutes, you can relax the muscles in your lower back/hips and chest/upper back with the tips provided in Chapters 18 and 19, respectively.

Other Tips to Rolling Right

Personally, I love to do my rolling in an outdoor setting. Firm grass, the right type of roller, and no ants are all I need. This setting provides me with plenty of space, a soft surface, and the sounds of nature. It also helps to be away from common distractions inside a busy house or workout room. And if you are like me and you find nature sounds, sights, and smells to be relaxing, outdoor rolling is a good way to create a relaxed mindset for effective rolling treatments.

PT NOTE

I recommend listening to relaxing music when rolling. My reasoning for this is based on the benefits of working with both the body and mind when enhancing your health. I've learned this with my patients, young and old, and with myself as an athlete. If the physical therapy focus is solely on the body and doesn't include the mind, the outcome will be subpar.

So, the benefits of relaxing music in a comfortable setting are huge. With your mind relaxed, your blood pressure low, your breathing rate low, and your body comfortable, your rolling experience will most certainly be more effective.

Conversely, trying to use a roller to unlock your lower back with loud music and loud kids is much more challenging. Let's be honest: Sometimes that's the exact setting we live in. So how do we get the most out of this setting?

Sometimes the solution is as simple as using earplugs and closing your eyes. By simply eliminating stressful noise and visuals from your setting for a mere five minutes, you can help your body and mind relax and unlock.

Think about it this way: Envision yourself driving down the highway with all your windows down, the radio blasting super loud, and you looking into the bright sun. Do you think that would be calming to your mind and body? No way!

Now think how your body and mind would respond when you roll up your windows, turn off the radio, and put on sunglasses. Much more relaxing, I'm sure.

You can use this same process if you eliminate stressful stimuli when rolling with the use of earplugs, closing your eyes, listening to relaxing music, and using soft lighting or a calming setting. It's all about preparing your body and mind to respond to the roller or roller ball. It's a lot easier to relax and knead cookie dough when it's warm than it is to do so when the cookie dough is cold. Your muscles respond in a similar fashion.

Padding and Pressure Relief

As you read through this book, you'll notice that staying comfortable while rolling is a common theme. By maintaining proper body position and minimizing predictable discomforts, the roller treatments will be quicker and more effective.

OUCH

Some of the roller treatments are uncomfortable. Applying pressure to locked muscles and trigger points is not what most people would call relaxing or calming. Mild to moderate pain can be expected for some of the treatments. But if you're in pain in other parts of your body because of contact with the ground or floor, that can be quickly corrected, as shown in Figure 3-2.

FIGURE 3-2: Many leg-rolling techniques require elbow padding to relax.

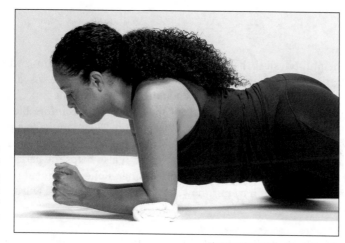

Photography by Haim Ariav & Klara Cu

Let's use your legs as an example: If you're rolling your legs to increase your quad flexibility and strength, it certainly won't help if you're in pain from bearing 50 percent of your body weight on the tip of your elbow. Such pain will increase both your heart rate and blood pressure. With a sudden increase in the blood flow and pressure in all your muscles, it makes it difficult for your four quad muscles to relax and respond to a roller treatment. So, a painful elbow, in this roller example, makes the objective of improving quad flexibility and function much harder to achieve.

The solution? Using a proper rolling technique and sufficient padding under sensitive areas of your body, as shown in Figure 3-3. This padding can come from fitness mats, yoga mats, carpet, grass, sand, pillows, rolled-up towels, or even wearable elbow or knee pads.

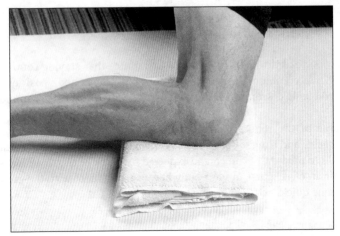

Photography by Haim Ariav & Klara Cu

FIGURE 3-3:
Knees are bony, so extra padding is helpful.

PT NOTE

A helpful physical therapy trick I've created is to keep my patients comfortable when my treatments are making them uncomfortable. As an example, if I'm working aggressively on their shoulder and causing them necessary pain, I want to ensure the other 95 percent of their body is as comfortable as possible. Certain physical therapy treatments are painful. They can make a patient feel worse before they get better. Explaining this to a patient in a simple manner will help the patient understand what they can expect. It also helps the patient gain confidence in their physical therapist or athletic trainer. Roller treatments can be an example of this process: It may hurt now, but if done properly, you will soon feel and move much better soon.

Let's use you as an example. Imagine you're feeling the pain of a roller ball burrowing into the back of your shoulder to unlock your posterior shoulder rotator cuff. Meanwhile, your hip is extremely painful from poor body posture and positioning against the wall. How relaxed do you feel? Do you feel your body and mind are primed for a great treatment?

Chances are your treatment results will suffer because other parts of your body, not being treated, are in pain. A simple footstool to elevate one of your feet or a verbal cue to correct your posture would increase your comfort and greatly enhance your treatment.

Chapter **4**
Caring for Your Roller

I n light of the recent COVID-19 pandemic, proper cleaning of your rollers has never been more important. The spreading of germs is never a good thing. When treating an injury or exercising on a roller, the last thing you want to do is spread an illness to or from a fellow roller.

With any exercise, sweating is inevitable. Sweat contains germs and bacteria along with the shedding of the outer layer of skin tissue. I share this not to gross you out but to remind you that the fluid left on your roller and floor after a, sweaty workout is not crystal-clear mountain-stream water.

Improving our hygiene and exercise equipment–cleaning practices needs to be a high priority for all of us. As the father of two young children, I'm learning that our personal cleaning habits, whether good or bad, are being watched and mimicked by our younger generation. Making those hygienic and illness-preventing actions strong is a must! With that in mind, this chapter shows you some easy ways to clean and care for your roller to ensure that it's safe to use and will last for years.

Cleaning Your Roller: Illness Prevention 101

Sharing rollers is never wise. Because of the obvious health concerns associated with sweating in public areas, having your own roller is a smart move. We have all seen rollers available in public places like gyms, fitness centers, and recreational fields. The physical therapist in me loves to see the free access to rollers everywhere. But the healthcare provider in me gets nervous when I see people sharing rollers in public places. The COVID-19 virus has opened our eyes to the ease with which a virus can be spread not only throughout our communities but around the world.

I recommend you treat your roller like your toothbrush: It's for you and you only.

Even if you are the only one to use your roller, cleaning the roller, as shown in Figure 4-1, and the rolling surfaces between each use is still highly recommended. It only makes sense if you think about it: Your roller's digging into your clammy skin across a dirty floor or mat while you breathe and sweat over everything. When you look at it that way, it's just common sense to clean the roller and the rolling surface before and after a rolling session.

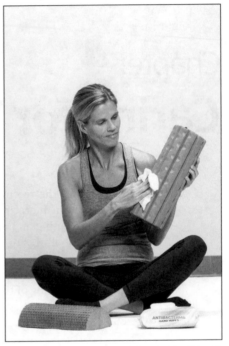

Photography by Haim Ariav & Klara Cu

FIGURE 4-1:
Thoroughly clean your roller before and after each use.

If you make this plan part of your normal routine, the cleaning will be very quick while you drastically reduce your risk of an illness.

Think about what an amazing combination you create through properly rolling on your own roller in your own home and using effective cleaning habits: reduced body pain, improved joint mobility, and improved muscle flexibility while reducing the risk of contracting an illness from others. Now compare that to an image of working out and sharing a roller in a public gym.

Many types of rollers are available, and their surface coverings vary greatly. Each roller surface differs in material, shape, size, and texture, as shown in Figure 4-2. The surface of each roller looks as varied as any landscape in the world: flat, high plains; smooth, rolling hills; short, steep foothills; and steep, jagged mountain cliffs.

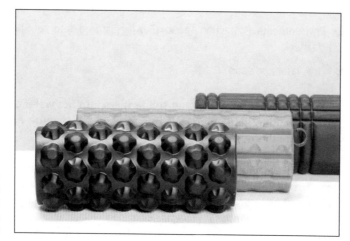

FIGURE 4-2:
Closeup view
of the different
surfaces on
rollers

Photography by Haim Ariav & Klara Cu

Each roller-covering material has different abilities to absorb or deflect fluids. Staying with the landscape analogy, each of the world's landscapes manages rainwater differently, as do the different roller surfaces with sweat and germs. Rain will gracefully glide off hard mountain rock, yet be absorbed quickly into soft farm soil. Sweat and germs will do the same, depending upon the type of material, creases, and openings found on the surface of a roller.

Identifying the proper cleaning solution for your roller is crucial. Carefully read the care and cleaning instructions for each roller. The cleaning details can be found in the shipping literature accompanying your roller or on the company's website.

PT NOTE

I mention this because some strong disinfectants commonly used for cleaning bathrooms and kitchen counters may discolor a roller. Personally, I thoroughly clean my rollers with strong, Environmental Protection Agency–approved products to ensure that my family and I are safe, even if the strong cleaning chemicals make my rollers look slightly tarnished and aged.

TIP

You can find more information at the Environmental Protection Agency (EPA) website (www.epa.gov).

Commercial disinfectants are the most effective products because they kill bacteria and virus microorganisms on surfaces. Follow all instructions on cleaning supplies to optimize their antimicrobial and antibacterial capabilities.

Here are some good options for cleaning your roller:

» Lysol disinfecting wipes

» Clorox disinfecting wipes

>> Environmental Protection Agency (EPA)-registered detergent-based spray cleaner

>> Hot water and soap

Completely submerging foam and solid rollers into hot water and soap is a quick and easy cleaning game plan, but this method will require extra time for your foam roller to thoroughly dry.

WARNING

Never submerge vibrating rollers, travel rollers, or any non-solid rollers into water. Cleaning electrical vibrating rollers requires special care to avoid damaging the electrical components inside the roller. Always defer to the manufacturer for specific care and cleaning instructions.

TIP

After an outdoor obstacle race or a sweaty roller session, I often bring my solid rollers into the shower with me. Hot water, soap, and a good scrubbing is a quick and easy way to initially clean my rollers post-race. When I arrive home, I break-out the "strong stuff" to thoroughly clean the rollers with EPA-approved wipes. I follow this by simply shaking the rollers out and placing them on a high shelf to air-dry.

Drying your rollers after cleaning is important. Never put your rollers in a clothes dryer or direct sunlight. Air-drying your rollers in a well-ventilated area on a clean surface is always the best option. Allow time and fresh air to dry all the small creases and valleys on the surface of the roller. Those areas are more prone to store bacteria, mildew, and mold. Being smart with your roller cleaning and drying routine helps you avoid turning your roller into a germ-filled petri dish.

Understanding What's Good and Bad About the Covering on Your Roller

It's no secret that I like to do off-road Spartan and obstacle course racing. Running and climbing in the woods is something I've loved to do since I first learned how to walk. As the youngest child of five, a mere one minute from claiming the number four spot proudly held by my twin brother, I'm pretty sure my very first step was into a muddy puddle.

The settings for my off-road obstacle course races are a far cry from my comfy living room or loaded workout room. Therefore, my pre-race and post-race rolling routines always take place in the mud, dirt, or grass.

At first, I arrived at these races with two or three of my favorite cloth-covered rollers. Needless to say, when I got home, my favorite rollers were super-dirty and stinky from rolling in smelly cow pastures, dusty fields, and swampy woods. I learned I needed a new race-day rolling game plan.

My plan: Switch to a harder, non-absorbing roller. Using a race-day roller with a harder, rubber, non-porous surface allows me to get my rollers wet and dirty in outdoor settings without the rollers absorbing fluids. I can now quickly rinse and properly clean my rollers with a super-strong cleaning material before and after my races.

OUCH

If it's super-muddy, my race-day roller is a 12-inch-long, 2-inch diameter piece of PVC pipe! It's the same white plastic piping you'd find connected to the under-side of your home kitchen sink. I wouldn't recommend this for the novice roller because rolling on a hard piece of PVC piping is about as subtle as a train wreck! With a perfect technique, it can unlock certain muscles, but it is very painful!

Here's a quick rundown of the pros and cons of various roller surfaces.

- » **Cloth/foam covering**
  - **Pro:** Softer, more comfortable.
  - **Con:** Absorbs sweat and fluid, harder to clean and dry, harder to roll on soft surfaces.
- » **Rubber, closed-cell, non-porous covering**
  - **Pro:** Easier to clean and dry, rolls easily on any surface.
  - **Con:** Moderately harder surface, more uncomfortable.
- » **Rubber surface with peaks and valleys**
  - **Pro:** More kneading and isolated treatments.
  - **Con:** More creases to hold germs, more difficult to clean.

Storing Your Roller

Hello. My name is Mike Ryan and I'm a roller addict. There, I said it. At least now I'm over the denial stage.

I own too many rollers and too many running shoes, according to my wife. She might be correct on the latter. Unlike my running shoes, I do use all my rollers.

I'm constantly experimenting with all my rollers and roller balls for different body parts, injuries, workouts, sports and even different stages of physical therapy for certain injuries.

As a roller addict with so many rollers, I've had to find effective ways to store them.

Most rollers are strong and sturdy. They can be used in almost any location and condition, rain or shine. They require very little maintenance. Let's be honest with each other: Rollers are our most loyal and trustworthy workout partners. They certainly make us feel better and help us perform at a much higher level whenever we call upon them. Just look at all these athletes having fun with their rollers in Figure 4-3.

But they still need some good ol' tender loving care.

REMEMBER

After cleaning your rollers following a treatment or workout, have a safe place to store them. My definition of a "safe place" is a location where the roller will not be damaged or infected by anything yucky.

With the number of high-tech materials and different designs in today's rollers, storing them in an excessively hot or cold setting can easily damage their integrity. It's easy to simply throw our roller into our gym bag and then toss the bag into the trunk of our car for the day as we stroll into our air-conditioned offices for a long day of work. Meanwhile, back in the 200°F trunk of our car, our loyal and loving friend, Robbie Roller, is melting. That just isn't right!

Both traveling rollers and vibrating rollers obviously have lots of moving parts and electronics to protect. Needless to say, if these types of rollers are exposed to excessive heat or cold, their damage can be permanent and expensive.

TIP

Treat your high-tech rollers and handheld massagers like you would your laptop. You wouldn't leave your laptop in the trunk of your hot car for eight hours. You wouldn't sweat on the keyboard of your laptop without cleaning between the keys. And you would certainly avoid leaving your laptop in the direct sunlight on the dashboard of your Tesla.

Let's get back to the "yucky" stuff. We've all learned a lot during the COVID-19 pandemic. Most of us quickly earned a doctorate degree in personal hygiene and hand washing. If we simply apply those same simple hygiene skills to our rollers, we'll take a big step in the right direction to keeping ourselves safer and healthier. After a roller treatment, we've all been guilty of using our workout towel to dry off our roller before throwing it into our germy workout bag, as shown in Figure 4-4. If you're "that guy or gal," you should feel really bad right about now.

Me: Guilty as charged.

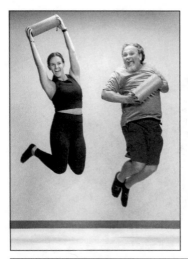

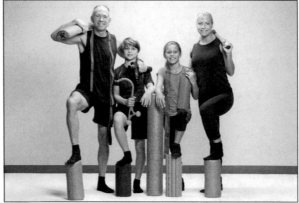

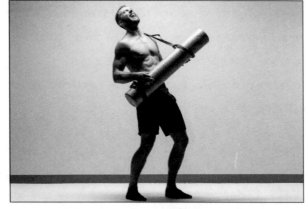

FIGURE 4-3:
Love thy roller,
in sickness and
in health.

Photography by Haim Ariav & Klara Cu

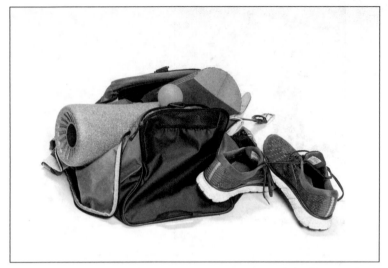

FIGURE 4-4:
A sad roller
haphazardly
thrown into a
dirty gym bag.

Photography by Haim Ariav & Klara Cu

TIP

Here are a few tips for safely storing your rollers between uses:

>> Boldly write your name or initials on your rollers to avoid accidentally sharing them with others.

>> Wipe your rollers and roller balls down with a Clorox or Lysol wipe before and after each use.

>> Allow your rollers to air-dry on a clean surface.

>> Don't put a roller in the dryer.

>> If travelling with a roller, place the roller in its own clean, waterproof bag.

>> Clean all handheld massager applicators as thoroughly as you do your rollers.

>> Don't expose your rollers to excessive heat or cold.

>> Have a place to store your rollers that is well ventilated and clean.

>> Store cleaning wipes with your rollers.

Chapter **5**
Roller Safety 101

Rollers can help you to prevent injuries, manage everyday aches and pains, and rehabilitate injuries. So, you don't want to get injured when you roll!

In this chapter, I share ways to avoid getting injured on a roller. This involves keeping the places where you roll safe. It also means learning who should avoid rollers because not everyone should be on a roller. Lastly, making a roller a positive and healthy tool for you means knowing what parts of your body should and should not be treated with a roller.

Assessing the Safety of Your Roller Rink

When rolling for a treatment or a workout, it's important to do it in a safe area. The space where you roll, or as I like to call it, your "roller rink," should be free of any hazards. Most hazards are obvious and clearly visible, but some of the most dangerous risks are harder to find.

Rolling surface

Make sure your rolling surface is well padded and consistent, as shown in Figure 5-1. Eliminate any localized slippery or sticky spots on your rolling surface. Ensure there are no small, sharp objects that can cause injury when a body part is placed on top of them. My home in Florida was reportedly built on an old World War I gun-firing range. I'm always finding pieces of glass in the dirt in my backyard. So when I'm rolling in my backyard grass, I scan for shiny glass and use a thicker mat to protect myself.

If you're rolling on an elevated deck or porch, it is wise to also make sure the underside of the entire rolling surface is well supported.

Your roller rink will go vertical as well, including on walls. Make sure the wall surface you will use is strong and supportive, as shown in Figure 5-2. The concern here is not the wall falling down; that will rarely happen. The typical concern is that parts of the wall surface may cave in. Poorly supported drywall or too much pressure on a hard roller ball can result in dents in the drywall. Having had the displeasure of fixing many of those drywall "potholes," trust me when I say that it's not a fun task.

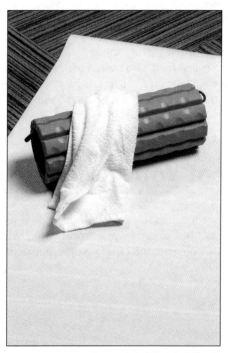

Photography by Haim Ariav & Klara Cu

FIGURE 5-1:
Padded and consistent surface for rolling.

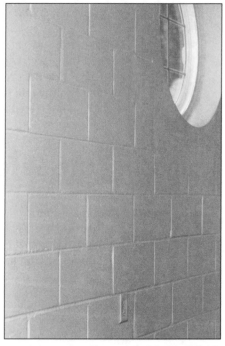

Photography by Haim Ariav & Klara Cu

FIGURE 5-2:
Solid wall with plenty of space to move and twist.

Roller rink real estate

Having enough floor and wall space to move in all four directions is important. A general rule of thumb, when appropriate, is to estimate how much floor surface area you need for your rolling treatment or workout, then double it. To start with, a 12-x-8 foot padded or carpeted space is sufficient for the average-sized person. Having worked with various professional athletes, I've noticed they need a much bigger plot of land to roll out, as shown in Figure 5-3.

When using a wall, it doesn't require much space. Typically, a 4-foot-wide wall is all you may need. The important thing is that you have clear access to the wall. Avoid chairs, tables, pictures, lights, or windows that you have to work around. You also need a stable floor with good traction as you move, bend, and twist against the wall during roller ball treatments.

Objects in the roller rink

Any object located inside the roller rink is a potential hazard. These objects may include furniture, workout equipment, smartphones, extraterrestrial creatures (just making sure you're awake), iPads, pets, or people.

Move objects out of your space before you start to roll. Clearing the needed space beforehand helps you relax during your treatment. Not having to think about banging into a table or a rock in the grass while you're rolling frees your mind to focus on breathing, maintaining perfect position, and unlocking tight muscles.

Objects positioned over the roller rink

It's easy to simply focus on the ground or the wall when rolling. Take some time to look for objects positioned above your roller rink for potential cranial collisions. These objects don't have to be hanging from the ceiling to be a potential problem for a roller. Hazards can include ceiling lights, tables, tree branches, pull-up bars, door handles, and open cabinet doors.

Objects landing in the roller rink

At first, this heading may sound far-fetched, but hear me out on this one. When rolling at home, you should avoid being injured by friendly fire. Friendly fire includes fast-walking spouses, high-energy kids, and love-seeking pets. In a gym or sports setting, keep a watchful eye open for projectile balls or fast-moving athletes.

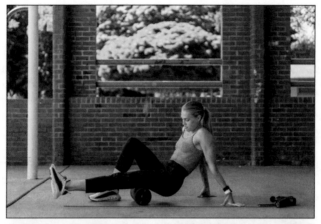

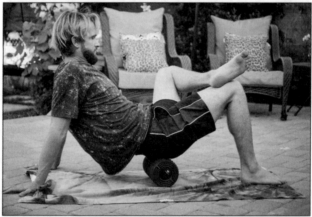

FIGURE 5-3: Rollers are used by athletes in every sport: Colleen Quigley (Olympian steeplechase runner), Brett Simpson (Head Coach, USA Olympic Surf Team), and Bec Wilcox (elite running coach).

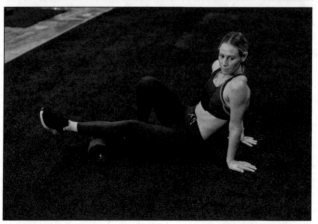

ROLLIN' ON THE ROAD

When travelling to races domestically and around the world, I often find myself packed into small hotel rooms or mobile RV homes the night before the race. As you probably know, hotel rooms in most countries are much smaller than those we commonly see in the United States. It makes rolling and stretching more challenging.

I ran in a long Spartan Beast Race in northern Montana in May of 2018. My wife, nine-year-old son, six-year-old daughter, and I packed into an RV mobile home for the adventure shown in the following photo. The limited space in the mobile home was less than ideal for my daily rolling and stretching routine.

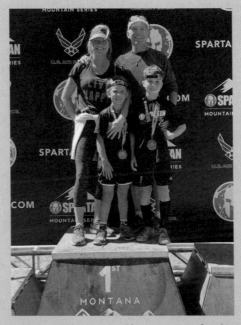

Photo courtesy of author

My solution: I took my show outside. My family knowingly shook their heads as I rolled in the Old Faithful parking lot at Yellowstone National Park; on a Wyoming dirt campsite next to a three-foot-high pile of snow; and in the wet, cold grass next to a flooded river in a town with the coolest of names; Anaconda, Montana.

Here's the cool thing about doing what I do. My kids love it! They both do Spartan Kids races and love to join me during my rolling sessions. Kids are so energetic and joyful about new "roller games" with their parents. My wife and I make it fun for our children by sharing healthy habits..

Who Should Not Be a Roller

Let's face it, rollers are not for everyone. Just like some exercise equipment doesn't work with some athletes, it's unwise and dangerous to force a roller session on someone who is physically or mentally not prepared to endure a roller treatment.

Rollers are very effective tools that enhance people's health, mobility, and lifestyle. But there are certain people, and injuries, where a roller should not be used. Continuing to hammer a round peg into a square hole is not a smart plan.

PT NOTE

Keeping others safe is a top priority for me. So sharing this message with those individuals who may become injured or worsen their present injury is important. Coordinating the details of your roller plans with your doctor is always a smart thing to do, just like you would do when starting a new exercise routine, diet, or medication.

WARNING

If you have any of the following conditions, get approval from your doctor before starting any roller treatment or workout:

>> Recent surgery

>> Pregnancy

>> Stroke

>> Open wounds

>> Cardiac pathologies

>> Total joint replacement

>> Vertigo/balance issues

>> Chronic pain

>> Neurological disorders/neuritis

>> Varicose veins

>> Diabetes

>> Fever

>> Skin disease

What Not to Roll

Not all body parts should be treated with a roller. In fact, there are a number of areas and types of tissue that need to be avoided. When it comes to using a roller, I relate it to one of my favorite humorous quotes:

If your only tool is a hammer, everything looks like a nail.

In other words, just because you have a roller doesn't mean you should use it on all your body parts nor all your aches and pains.

WARNING

Certain parts of your body will not respond to a roller. Worse, using the roller on certain types of tissue will cause excessive pain and injury. For example, using a hard, small roller over the funny bone, the ulnar nerve on the inside of the elbow joint, can injure the nerve. When this happens, it results in prolonged numbness, pain, and weakness in your ring finger and small finger.

Another example of parts of your body to avoid when rolling is the lateral hip. The official medical term for the "lateral hip bone" is the greater trochanter of the femur or thigh bone. It's the bony landmark located between your front and back pants pockets. This is a hard, bony ridge that would not respond well to a roller. A big concern here is that this ridge is covered by a thin bursa. The role of the greater trochanter bursa is to provide a smooth cushion for the tendons gliding back and forth across the bony ridge for both hips. So, running a roller over the bony hip bone could inflame the bursa, leaving you with a painful and slow-healing bursitis.

Here are some other *roller no-fly zones* that you should avoid:

>> Bone

>> Nerves

>> Bursa

>> Breasts (female)

>> Areas not approved for physical therapy by a treating physician

>> Open wounds

>> Wounds containing infection, stitches, or staples

>> Wounds less than four weeks removed from infection, stitches, or staples

>> Areas where the pressure of the roller results in shooting pins and needles and tingling pain from the treatment site

>> Areas where the discomfort from the contact site is excessive or prolonged

PT NOTE

Knowing the difference between "good pain" and "bad pain" is important to stay healthy. When rolling, *good pain* is when you feel your muscles relax and your joint range of motion increase (see Figure 5-4). It may still be uncomfortable, but the pain is accompanied by a "warm flush," a sense of your muscles and fascia relaxing and lengthening.

Meanwhile, *bad pain* is sharp and tightening, as shown in Figure 5-5. While the pain is excessive, you notice your muscles and fascia tightening, in a protective manner resulting in a loss of joint range of motion.

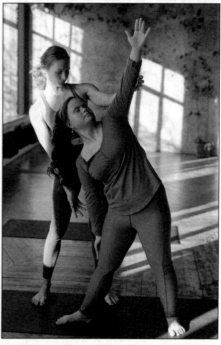

Source: Photo by Cliff Booth from Pexels

FIGURE 5-4:
"Good pain" accompanies post-rolled muscles, tendons and fascia relaxing in a healthy manner.

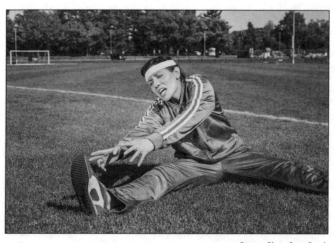

FIGURE 5-5:
All-too-familiar bad pain!

Source: Photo from Pexels

Avoiding Injury on a Roller

PT NOTE

There is an important quote that I share with young physical therapists, athletic training students, and my patients. The quote seems overly simple, but its value is very powerful. Having worked for 26 years as a physical therapist for the NFL, I can tell you the line between aggressive physical therapy and re-injuring an athlete is very thin. This quote highlights the difference between the two sides of that line.

If you can't make the patient better, at least don't make them worse.

Think about this quote for a moment. Putting yourself in the position of the patient, you want to be as aggressive as possible to get back as close to 100 percent as quickly as possible, *but* you don't want to cross the line to get injured and regress. Being realistic, you also don't want to baby yourself or wrap yourself in bubble wrap so as not to get injured. If you're an athlete, you will push yourself hard to optimize your outcome.

REMEMBER

This wise motto applies to you for both roller self-treatments and your workouts. When it comes to using a roller to improve your health, the last thing you want to do is to create an injury.

The most common way of getting injured on a roller is to roll over a sensitive body part, as noted in the previous section. Rolling in a *roller no-fly zone* can produce pain and possibly damage the tissue. It doesn't take a rocket scientist to realize that anything you do to injure your tissue and produce sharp or intense pain should never be part of your game plan.

REMEMBER

Another risk factor for a roller injury is poor body position. When rolling a body part, as I describe in Parts 2, 3, and 4 of this book, a stable and healthy body position is mandatory. In contrast, putting your body in an awkward or contorted position while rolling can result in an injury. The position shown in Figure 5-6a puts too much pressure and strain on the lower lumbar spin and sacrum. Figure 5-6b shows an excessive low back extension that overloads the junction where the bottom two lumbar vertebra rest on top of the sacrum. (This segment of the spine is referred to as the L4-L5 and L5 – S1 disc spaces. Over 75 percent of lumbar disc injuries take place in these two joints.) Finally, applying localized pressure on the side or front of the neck with a roller ball as shown in Figure 5-6c makes important structures such as your nerves, blood vessels, lymph nodes, and windpipe vulnerable to injury.

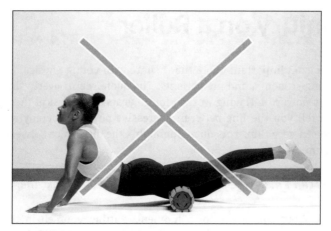

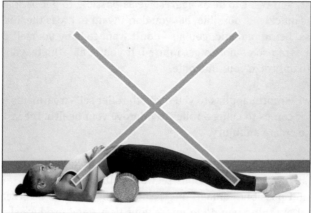

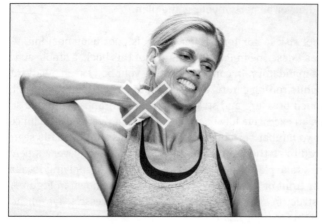

FIGURE 5-6:
Examples of
dangerous
rolling
treatments.

Photography by Haim Ariav & Klara Cu

In addition, being in an uncomfortable and improper position is not conducive to total body relaxation. That, in turn, will produce sub-par results during your rolling treatments.

Table 5-1 shows some examples.

TABLE 5-1   ## Potential Injuries When Rolling With Poor Posture

Body Part Treated	Common Error	Potential Injury
Legs	Twisted spine	Low back pain
Posterior shoulder	Excessive internal rotation	Shoulder impingement syndrome
Anterior shoulder	Prolonged pressure on long-head of the biceps tendon	Chronic tendonitis
Mid-spine	Excessive neck extension	Neck pain
Elbow	Excessive pressure on the lateral elbow joint line	Tennis elbow
Calf	Excessive pressure on the calf muscle scar tissue	Chronic calf pain
Legs	Insufficient elbow padding	Elbow bursitis
Arch	Excessive pressure on the heel bone	Plantar fasciitis

REMEMBER

Simply stated: Rolling the *right* muscles, with the *right* posture, avoiding the *wrong* body parts, with the *right* breathing, with the *right* technique, will produce the *right* results!

Here are some tips to help you avoid being injured using a roller:

>> Always use proper roller techniques, period.

>> Start slow and learn how each part of your body responds to different rollers, pressure, and techniques.

>> Know the difference between "good pain" and "bad pain."

>> Perform a quick 30-second march/squat/arm circles/twist routine before and immediately after you roll to answer the question: "Did my treatment make me better or worse?"

>> Listen to your body. It's much smarter than we give it credit for.

>> Know your roller "no-fly zones" and respect their boundaries.

>> Keep the discomfort levels associated with roller treatments or workouts between mild and moderate.

2

Rolling the Right Way

Knowing when and when not to use a roller

Properly preparing and warming up your body for a roller treatment

Using your roller effectively by working *with* your muscles

Accelerating your post-workout recovery using your rollers

Chapter **6**
Timing Is Everything: When and When Not to Roll

This chapter will cover the importance of proper roller timing. As with every piece of exercise and physical therapy equipment, knowing *when* to use them is just as important as knowing *how* to use them.

There are so many factors when it comes to rolling: The type of roller, the size of the roller, the length of the treatment, the type of warming up for the roller, how you manage the pain of the treatment, and how you assess the benefits of the treatment. So it only makes sense that the timing of the treatment is important as well.

There are times when a roller can be your BFF; Best Friend Forever. The roller timing issue is important because it will keep you safe while allowing you to optimize the many benefits of a roller. Simply stated: Smart timing on a roller will help you decrease your risk and increase your results.

REMEMBER

As you gain experience with different rollers and enhance your ability to truly listen to your body's response to the rollers, you will naturally start adjusting your roller timing and techniques.

Knowing When to Roll

Rolling is just a part of our wellness plan. Most of us use a roller and stretching to enhance our body's ability to move better with less effort. If we and the rollers do our job well, our muscles have more flexibility, our joints have more mobility, and our body has less pain.

REMEMBER

The quote, "If a little is good, a lot is better," does not apply to rollers. Many rehabilitation tools and instruments used by physical therapists and athletic trainers can be overused if not properly scheduled. When it comes to mastering the art of successful roller rehab, the timing of *when* and *how* to use the roller is a mandatory skill.

THE HAMMER

An important machine breaks down in a big factory. No one working at the factory can fix the machine, so a special mechanical engineer is called in to get the machine up and running.

The engineer spends an hour walking around the broken machine in a deep trance. He continues to look, listen, and feel the machine with immense concentration. He crawls around the machine with slow, precise movements. Finally, he pulls a small hammer from his massive toolbox, and whacks the machine with a single swing using laser-like precision. The machine immediately starts up and runs as smoothly as it did the first day they turned it on.

When the company receives the invoice for the 60 minute service call by the engineer, it reads as follows:

Whacking a machine with a hammer: $5

Knowing when and where to whack the machine with the hammer: $495

Total: $500

I'm sharing this hammer story with you to emphasize an important point. Grinding away on a roller with no treatment plan is painful and ineffective. But knowing *when* and *where* to place the roller, much like the engineer did with his hammer, results in a comfortable and effective treatment.

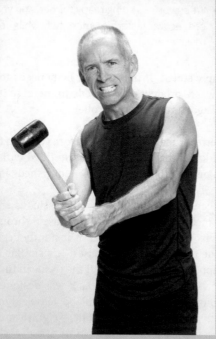

Photography by Haim Ariav & Klara Cu

Best times to roll

There are certain times when a roller will optimize your body's ability to do its job. For example,

>> When your body feels stiff and tight, it's a good time to use a roller.

>> When you feel a knot or trigger point in a muscle, but you know this is not a new muscle strain, it's a good time to use a roller.

>> If you're getting ready to start a physically demanding activity such as exercising, working in the yard, playing with the kids, or carrying heavy luggage through an airport, it's a good time to use a roller.

>> When you're in the middle of an activity, workday, workout, or project and a muscle knot or "creak" decides to make itself known in one of your muscles, it's a good time to use a roller.

>> After a hard endeavor when your muscles are ready for a well-earned nap, it's a good time to use a roller.

>> When you're getting ready for bed and you want to relax your muscles so they can recover faster and more fully while you sleep, it's a good time to use a roller.

REMEMBER

Simply stated: If part of your body needs to be less bound down, needs to reduce its waste products, and needs to increase its supply of good, oxygen-rich blood, it's a good time to use a roller.

TIP

A perfect time for a roller is before you plan to put a group of your muscles to work. You know that a relaxed muscle filled with a consistent inflow of healthy blood will perform better. A mobile, nourished, and strong muscle is a happy muscle.

We can never forget about our fascia, as shown in Figure 6-1. A roller improves the mobility of the ever-active fascia throughout the body. When the tension on and from fascia is reduced, it instantly decreases the restrictive stress on all the tissue the fascia encompasses. It's similar to unraveling duct tape that is tightly wrapped around a thigh. All the tissue in the front, inside, back, and outside of the thigh is now free to move as it was designed to move. In addition to the muscles throughout the thigh, the blood vessels, lymphatic vessels, nerves, tendons, scar tissue, and the fascia itself have significantly more mobility. And, when it comes to these very important types of tissue, each of them can now do their jobs much more effectively.

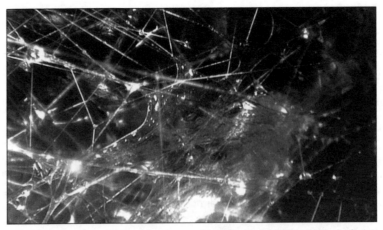

FIGURE 6-1:
Inside look at
fascia.

J.C. Guimberteau M.D/ENDOVIVO Video Productions

Once again using the example of duct tape tightly wrapped around a thigh, imagine how difficult it is for blood to flow properly through fascia-restricted areas when exercising at a very high level. The nerves also become entrapped and sensitive because of the excess pressure. I often find nerve entrapments to be a common source of my patients' chronic pain.

With all the previously noted benefits of rolling, it shouldn't come as a surprise to learn that rolling is also a valuable tool for post-activity recovery.

Think about it this way: Following a hard activity or busy day at work, your muscles need to rid themselves of all their toxins. They need to get the bad stuff out and the good stuff in. A roller is a perfect tool to improve the efficiency of the lymphatic system to drain off those toxins and waste products from the muscles and surrounding tissue.

Another roller-recovery benefit involves the circulatory system. Relaxing muscles and fascia will improve the body's ability to pump fresh blood, rich with oxygen, water, electrolytes, and calories, to hungry muscles. Tight and bound-down muscles are more likely to cramp when they become dehydrated. We spend a considerable amount of our time, effort, and money maintaining a healthy diet and hydration plan. But if our muscles are too tight and restricted, we may be limiting our body's ability to effectively transport those calories and fluids to our hard-working and hungry muscles.

Optimal times to rock and roll with a roller or roller ball:

» Pre-morning coffee

» Post-morning coffee

» Pre-workout

» During workout breaks

» Long days at your desk (see Figure 6-2a)

» During work breaks

» When you need a midday nap or a cold cup of water thrown in your face to wake you up, and neither one is an available option

» During long car rides (see Figure 6-2b and c)

» Post–long car rides

» Post-exercise

» While travelling

» While watching TV at home with your family

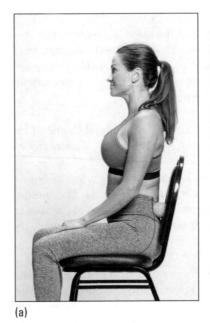

(a)

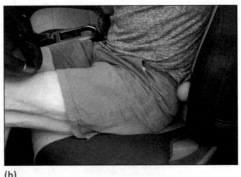

(b)

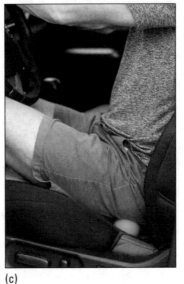

(c)

FIGURE 6-2:
Roller ball used
for hip and
low back pain
when sitting.

Pre-sleep rolling tips

I'm a big fan of using a roller before I go to bed. It helps me unwind from a busy day and removes tension and tightness in my spine and extremities. My pre-sleep rolling routine is my secret weapon to accelerate my recovery while I sleep. It allows me to wake up earlier and feel fresher for my daily pre-sunrise workouts.

At the risk of sounding like a crazy man, I want you to take one minute to be super-creative with me. Imagine yourself living inside your thigh muscles (Figure 6-3) — strange, I know, but stay with me. At the end of a long, busy day, you (thigh muscles) feel super-tight and bound down. You have lots of gunk and stagnant fluid just hanging around you. Minimal blood is moving in or out of you, because you're all cinched down with yards of fascia wrapped around you and every muscle in your leg. You, the muscle, is now short and tight from sitting all day and you haven't been stretched in nine or more hours! This sucks!

But after a quick roller treatment, the tight tension is gone, and you can finally breathe — you're alive again! As you're tucked into bed for a solid eight hours of sleep, you and your neighborhood muscles are purring with pleasure. It's like someone just opened the plug at the bottom of the bathtub in your muscle. All the bad gunk is flushing out of all your corners, as yummy, fresh blood effortlessly flows in. Life is good again.

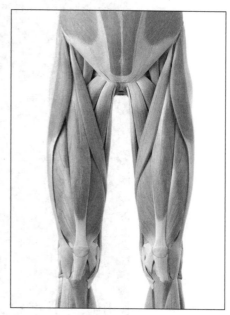

SciePro/Shutterstock

FIGURE 6-3:
The busy neighborhood of the thigh.

Now, come back to reality.

Imagine the stark difference you would see and feel inside the thigh muscles before and after a rolling treatment. Just think how happy and relaxed those sleeping muscles and fascia will be in the morning!

Instead of those leg muscles having to work hard both supporting your body and removing muscle waste products *uphill* against gravity, the freshly rolled legs and fascia are now relaxed and laying horizontally in bed. Now the legs can easily absorb fresh in-flowing blood from the heart via the arteries and effectively remove toxins and waste products via the lymphatic system (shown in Figure 6-4) and veins.

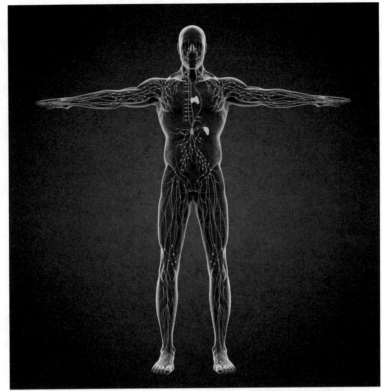

FIGURE 6-4:
The most ignored, but important, system in the human body: the lymphatic system.

STARTING AND ENDING THE DAY THE RIGHT WAY

I roll my body every night before I go to bed and as soon as I get up in the morning. I find my pre-sleep rolling routine is a wonderful way to relieve the tension in my muscles, tendons, and fascia. I sleep more deeply and I move less. When I look at my sleep technology data thanks to my Select Comfort bed and my Garmin watch, I consistently have healthier rapid eye movement (REM) cycles and less movement on the nights that I have a strong rolling session prior to bedtime! I'm not surprised by that objective data because my body has demonstrated the rewards of my rolling routine, but seeing those numbers is a huge motivator for me to stay the course with my pre-sleep routine.

Another reward for my pre-bedtime rolling routine, shown in the figure, comes in the morning. As I mentioned, I also roll when I first wake up. (Confession: My 5 a.m. pre-rolling warm-up is minimal.) The morning roll session is so much easier and less painful when it follows a strong pre-bedtime rolling session the night before! Think about that for a moment: If I do my job of rolling properly at 9:30 or 10 p.m. the night before, my muscles are looser, less painful, and more flexible seven hours later!

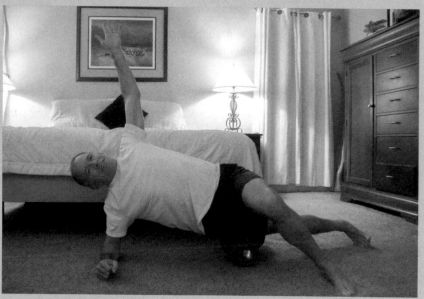

Photography by Haim Ariav & Klara Cu

Knowing When *Not* to Roll

Knowing when *not* to roll is as important as knowing when to roll. As I explain in Chapter 5, using a roller on certain injuries or body parts can be detrimental. Some of this is common sense. Being smart with our rollers helps us avoid creating an injury or making an injury worse.

Listening to a painful injury

Our bodies are extremely smart. But sometimes we're not smart enough to listen to them. Now is a perfect time to learn to trust your "gut feelings" when it comes to your body. In this day and age when technology appears to be king, it's easy to get away from our less-subjective and less-visible body and mind feedback. Too often, we rely on smartphones, apps, computers, videos, and experts to get our health and wellness advice. I want to change that.

It's time that we all go "old school" by improving our communication skills with our own bodies. Our bodies give us tons of information per second. We will become smarter and healthier when we improve our ability to listen to those messages.

No one knows your body as well as you do. That is a powerful statement that needs repeating: "No one — not your doctor, not your spouse, not your personal trainer, not your mirror, not your bathroom scale, not your best friend — knows your body as well as you do."

Pain management versus avoidance of pain

Now let's shift to working with your body when managing pain or an injury. News flash: Using a roller can be uncomfortable, if not painful. So, when you move a roller over a body part that is painful at rest, it's an uncomfortable experience. Listening to that painful body part is an important skill we all need to improve on. Some people's quest is to avoid any and all pain. That is rarely possible when it comes to being active and even growing old. A smarter and healthier quest should be learning how to wisely manage pain, not avoid it.

Pain is just another message from the body to the brain. It's usually a loud message, that is true, but it's still just a message. In Chapter 5, I differentiated between "good pain" and "bad pain." This is another example of why that skill is so important. If a roller treatment, stretch, strengthening exercise, cardio drill, or workout routine makes your pain less severe, less frequent, or of a shorter duration, then it is good for you. Conversely, if anything you are doing is making your pain worse, common sense tells you to discontinue that part of your routine.

The last thing you want to do is make a sore body part or injury worse with your treatments. But knowing how your body is responding to your routine is the key. For example, if your shoulder is suffering from an impingement syndrome causing pain in the front and outside of your shoulder, you will learn how to roll the muscles of your posterior shoulder rotator cuff. If done properly, your anterior and lateral shoulder pain will be much improved, but your posterior shoulder will be more painful. So, your injury pain (bad pain) is better, but the treatment site pain (good pain) is worse. This is where you need to understand that you are not seeking the complete absence of pain but, instead, seeking the healthy alternative of significantly reducing your "bad pain."

I hope you're grasping my pain management concept.

Seeking to understand and be understood: The mind-body connection

TIP

To help reinforce this point, I want to piggyback on a great quote from Stephen Covey's best-selling book, *The 7 Habits of Highly Effective People: Seek first to understand, then to be understood.*

Seek first to understand your body:

>> What does my body like or dislike?

>> What helps my body move better or worse?

>> What are my body's strengths and weaknesses?

>> Does my body run better on carbohydrates, proteins, or fats?

>> What helps my body sleep better or worse?

Then seek to understand your mind:

>> What are my motivators and goals?

>> What are my fears?

>> How tough or weak am I?

>> What is my mind's Achilles heel?

Another amazing skill our super-smart body has is to protect itself from bad pain. For example, if you're aggressively rolling a painful posterior shoulder injury but demonstrating poor posture on the roller, your body may respond with an upper-back muscle spasm. This is the body's attempt to protect the shoulder girdle and spine from injury.

The human body is focused on protecting itself before it worries about performing at a high level. This is why I developed the concept of "working *with* the body, not *against* the body." If your social media–driven ego is focused on a hefty outcome for which your body is not properly prepared, your body and mind will not cooperate.

Therefore, listening to instead of ignoring a sore body part or injury is always a smart move. Your body will tell you what it needs *more* of and what it needs *less* of. This may include more or less rest, roller treatments, stretching, posture exercises, core exercises, fluids, sleep, stretching, electrolytes, manual therapy, and healthy calories.

The roller routine for your sore body part or injury can be easily altered by using a softer roller, less pressure, a longer warm-up, and eliminating active motion during the treatment. I will discuss the progressions and changes within your roller program later in this book.

Rolling warning signs you should never ignore

WARNING

There are a few warning signs from your body that indicate you may be rolling too aggressively. These warning signs should never be ignored:

>> Intense localized pain

>> Intense pain extending away from the roller pressure point

>> Involuntary muscle spasm above, at, or below the roller pressure point

>> Numbness, pins and needles, burning, or shooting pain at or below the roller pressure point

>> An involuntary, blood-curdling scream worthy of a late-night horror movie

>> Chest pains, pain down your upper-left arm, severe shortness of breath, or a combination of these

>> Sudden rashes, hot flashes, or fever

>> Dizziness, changes in balance, or blurred vision

>> Joint catching, shifting, or locking

Chapter **7**

Warming Up Your Body for the Roller

At work or play, getting more done in less time is a common goal for us all. And that's one of my favorite traits of rollers. They're easy to use and they work fast — if your body is prepped for the roller.

Most of us, myself included, want to skip the warm-up to spend more time working out. It's easy to blame that attitude on our busy schedules or long To-Do lists. The truth is that most people see little value in the warm-up part of their wellness plan. But when it comes to using a roller to literally steamroll your muscles, blood vessels, fascia, tendons, nerves, lymphatic vessels, adhesions, and skin with an aggressive treatment, it's imperative to prepare all of those body tissues for the onslaught that follows.

In this chapter, I show you how to properly warm up your body and mind to maximize your roller sessions.

Preparing Your Entire Body for the Roller

When the human body experiences pain, even in one small, isolated area, the entire body is impacted. Conversely, when pain is eliminated, it's "party time!" When the body is pain-free, it instantly functions better. So, when preparing for a roller treatment, it's important for you to "take the blinders off" and thoroughly assess your body for restrictions at, above, and below the treatment site.

One reason why it's important to prepare both above and below the treatment site is that many skeletal muscles in the human body cross multiple joints. Therefore, treating those muscles will impact joints above and below the muscle belly. Rapid increases in joint ranges of motion above and below the unlocked muscle is your goal.

TIP

I share with my athletes three simple questions to ask themselves prior to a roller treatment. If they can answer "Yes" to all three questions, they're "ready to rock and roll!"

>> Am I sweating?

>> Is my heart rate at least 25 beats higher than it was when I woke up this morning?

>> Can I get into and out of the proper rolling positions without sounding or looking like I'm 90 years old?

Here are some examples of warm-up activities to do before roller treatments:

>> Roller stick

>> Handheld massager

>> Low intensity cardio exercise. See Figure 7-1

>> Body massage

>> Biking

>> Power walking

>> Dancing

>> Elliptical trainer

>> Swimming

>> Shadow boxing

>> Relaxing in a hot tub or taking a shower

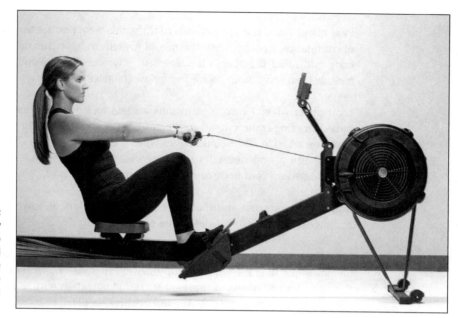

FIGURE 7-1:
Low-intensity
exercise to
increase blood
flow into the
tissue to be
treated with
the roller.

Photography by Haim Ariav & Klara Cu

Warming Up Your Mind Before Rolling

"Warming up my mind? Does this guy want me to use a roller on my brain?!"

No. Your brain is safe. For now.

What I mean by "warming up your mind" is preparing your brain, your nerves, and your attitude for a roller treatment. Roller treatments are a very effective way to unlock muscles. However, they are also often uncomfortable, strenuous, and challenging to say the least. Few people will confuse roller treatments with a relaxing massage at a plush Hawaiian oceanfront spa.

PT NOTE

Wrapping your head around the objectives and the techniques associated with roller treatments is the first step. Keeping your "eye on the prize" is a helpful tip for every roller treatment. What I mean by that is focusing on the exact outcome you expect from every treatment. For example, let's say you're rolling your chest muscle because of a painful shoulder impingement. For this treatment, it would be helpful for you to visualize yourself brushing your hair afterwards. This bright and colorful cranial movie will help you endure the discomfort of the roller treatment. By visualizing yourself brushing your hair with a pain-free shoulder, you're warming up your mind and body for success.

I ask my physical therapy patients to think this way, but not to create a false sense of confidence. Instead, I ask them, and myself, to have this mindset to join their body and mind together. All successful physical therapy and exercise routines include hard work, both above and below the neck.

I get upset when I hear a victorious athlete look in the camera and say mentally degrading comments like: "I can't believe I won!" or "I never expected to be here!" or "THEY said I could never win!" Don't be that guy or gal! Never doubt your abilities. And never let someone else's negativities or doubt occupy your brain regarding your body or mind for even a split second.

Don't get me started on this topic because I have lots of powerful examples and insight on the hidden abilities of the human mind.

TIP

Visualize successful roller treatments. See yourself pain-free. Expect to be active and strong. And share your very optimistic roller visions with others. We take on the attitudes and habits of those we surround ourselves with. Fill your inner circle with positive, caring, supportive, and healthy people.

Active + Healthy = Happy

Pop quiz time: If you were preparing to play in a championship game in, say, any of the major college sports (football, basketball, hockey, soccer, wrestling, or track), what is the ONE thing you would be 100 percent guaranteed to face in that game?

Seeing the very wide range of sports listed here, that's a very bold question, wouldn't you say? With those different sports, there's no commonality with the ball, weather, scoring, number of players, temperatures, footwear, playing surface, or injuries.

Any guesses?

My answer: *Pain.*

Think about it. With all those sports being played at a high level against strong competition, some degree of pain is the only common factor.

PT NOTE

That's why I find it peculiar that most sports use practice time to prepare their athletes for all potential challenges they will face in their next game. Meanwhile, they spend very little time even discussing a game plan for the only known obstacle they are guaranteed to face: pain. I love the topic of pain because it possesses so much complexity, depending on which angle you look at it.

Pain can be a funny thing. Some people go to extreme lengths to avoid any and all pain. Personally, I practice the art of understanding and managing pain in both my sports and my profession. Warming my mind up for my physical therapy treatments includes preparing my body and mind to manage the inevitable pain to follow.

REMEMBER

This doesn't mean you're preparing your mind for a life-altering pain-fest. It simply means your mind understands some discomfort is soon to follow. Meanwhile, your mind is calm because it understands the arriving discomfort is a form of "good pain." Your confident mind also understands that the manageable discomfort you are inflicting on your body is a small price to pay for the compounded-interest benefits coming from your roller treatments.

Getting the Rolling Site Ready for Contact

"The *Eagle* has landed" was the famous Neil Armstrong quote when the Apollo 11 Lunar Module *Eagle* first landed on the moon on July 20, 1969. When your roller module first touches down on your body, with presumably much less international fanfare than Armstrong experienced, make sure your landing site is properly prepared.

If you follow the two previous warm-up steps, both your body and your mind will be ready for the treatment. This third step focuses solely on the localized area being treated. This is where you probably have pain, trigger points, adhesions, scar tissue, or restrictions. It is the area that needs fixing, so to speak.

TIP

A simple way to look at this process is that you're getting the local tissue warmer and moving more. When you increase the mobility and blood flow into the skin, fascia, muscle, blood vessels, lymphatic vessels, nerves, and adhesions, the metabolism of those cells quickly increases. By waking up or "turning on" all those tissue cells prior to the treatment, you ensure that the entire area is better prepared to respond positively to the roller. This helps you take a huge stride towards returning your tissues back to their normal, pain-free function.

PT NOTE

A proper warm-up will result in the following physiological changes in your body:

>> Increased blood flow

>> Increased heart rate

>> Increased tissue temperature

>> Increased muscle metabolism

>> Increased sweat rate

>> Increased lymphatic drainage

>> Increased muscle strength

>> Improved nerve conduction

REMEMBER

Here are a few helpful takeaways:

>> The warm-up will increase the benefits of your roller treatment.

>> You need to prepare your entire body, not just the roller treatment sites.

>> The best warm-up involves the body, mind, and everything in between.

Chapter **8**

Work *With* Your Muscles, Not *Against* Them

I spent 26 wonderful years working as an athletic trainer and physical therapist in the National Football League (NFL), as seen in Figure 8-1. During that time, I became an expert at managing trauma. I watched dozens of violent collisions on every single play of every practice during those years, which included 533 NFL games. Just think how many times those professional football players' bodies slammed into opposing players, their own protective equipment, the rock-hard football, and the ground. The numbers are staggering.

Looking at the NFL trauma issue helps to demonstrate how resilient the human body is to stress. Imagine the stress an agile, 330-pound professional football player puts on his legs just running and changing direction on a hard field at, say, 13 miles per hour while wearing up to 25 pounds of protective equipment. And that doesn't include any contact or collisions. This example is just a big man running and changing directions. Professional football players are large, strong human beings; the largest NFL player I ever rehabbed as a physical therapist weighed 404 pounds.

Needless to say, those elite athletes need very strong and flexible muscles to perform at a very high level. If those same muscles are injured or don't function optimally for any reason, their performance suffers. It's common sense, but if an expensive professional athlete's performance drops off, they are at a high risk of being fired, or "cut" as they say in the NFL, by their team. That's a big deal. The average NFL player's salary in 2019 was $3,200,000, but if they're cut, most of those salaries immediately drops to $0.

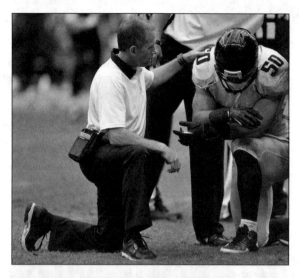

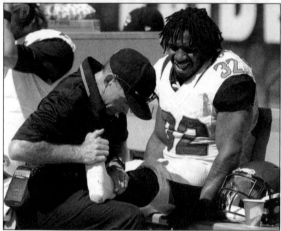

Rick Wilson

FIGURE 8-1:
The author
working in the
NFL.

This is why I developed my "work *with* your muscles, not *against* them" philosophy for my athletes and patients.

PT NOTE

As a physical therapist, when I visualize how my patients' bodies work, I ask myself, "What do these muscles need to be strong, flexible, and responsive?" By doing this, I'm comparing how I know their muscles, tendons, and joints are working with how I know they *should* be working. I understand this is a very deep philosophical and anatomical concept for you to understand. Simply stated, it's more like you're literally putting yourself into the muscle and understanding how to make that muscle achieve its optimal performance instead of battling with the muscle, and trying to force it to do what you think is best.

By using this approach with someone in pain, and working with the muscle, I help the patient and the muscle gain more confidence when contracting and stretching at their own pace. The patient then controls the pace of the roller treatments, stretches, and exercises. No matter what the exercise or drill is, it starts slow; even walking is fine. I then watch the patient's confidence grow. Their silent fear which naturally makes them think, "ohhh will this move hurt and reinjure the muscle?" is soon eliminated.

You may be asking yourself, "I'm not a professional football player, so will this approach work for me?" To answer that question, I want you to take a trip with me, back in time. You're exerting yourself during a sweaty workout, or maybe you're working in your yard. The only problem: You're sore and in pain. It certainly isn't fun, is it? The pain is concerning, of course, but the questions of *why* you are in pain and *whether* your active lifestyle is making your painful injury worse you're chipping away at your confidence. Your pain is a major source of stress for you. It is making you resent your aging body, and it is making you feel old.

But now I offer you a simple and inexpensive set of tools — rollers — to help you quickly control a majority of your muscle and soft-tissue tightness and pain.

In this chapter, you'll discover my "secret sauce" to successful rolling treatments: my Five Ryan Rolling Rules. These rules will be used every time you roll. You'll quickly learn these five rules will accelerate both your ability to unlock your tight muscles and eliminate soft tissue pain. So buckle up and grab your pen and notepad because you're about to become a smarter, healthier, and more mobile athlete!

My Five Ryan Rolling Rules

Here are my five rolling rules, your game plan to help you master the art of muscle rolling:

>> Align the spine

>> Breathe

>> Slow your roll

>> Seek and destroy trigger points

>> Move the muscle

I've molded, tweaked, and refined these rules over the past 25 years with thousands of athletes, young and old, including myself. As my wife, a fellow Ironman triathlete, will attest, I'm on a hard roller every morning before the sun rises and every night before I go to bed (see Figure 8-2).

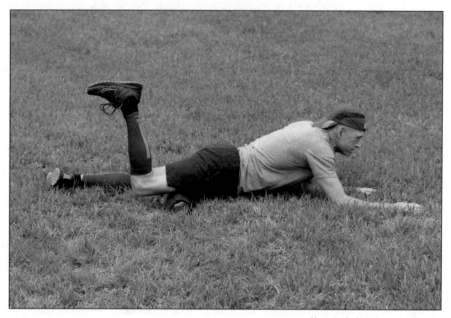

FIGURE 8-2: The author practicing what he preaches.

Anyone who knows me will tell you I'm an energetic and always-moving kind of guy. At least six days per week, I'm out of bed, ready to work out by 5:30 a.m. Most people are surprised to learn I don't drink coffee, and I'm constantly asked, "How do you get up so early and exercise so hard without coffee?"

My answer is always the same: "My rollers."

Why rollers? My answer is based on two truths about a hard roller at 5:30 a.m.:

>> **It hurts.** Unlike coffee, which slowly brings your senses to life, pain hits you in the face like a shovel! One moment you're yawning, rubbing the sleep from your eyes, and 12 seconds later your quads are screaming, your heart rate doubles, and your mind snaps to attention.

>> **It works.** Rollers loosen up everything between the skin and the bones. A roller saves you warm-up time by accelerating your body's ability to increase muscle flexibility, blood flow, and joint range of motion.

Align the spine

Think of aligning the spine as using proper posture on the roller. Sure, you're moving and bending your body as you unlock muscles, but you don't want that motion to put your spine in a bad position. All your treatments can be performed on the floor or on the wall, with perfect technique, without compromising the support or health of your spine.

REMEMBER

You never want to create a new injury or worsen an existing injury when you're rolling. The act of rolling will put your body in some unusual positions. Those positions can add stress to other parts of your body, especially your neck and lower back. Properly aligning your spine for the entire treatment is important enough to make my top five rolling rules.

To protect your spine — from your pelvis to your skull — while rolling, I strongly suggest you maintain proper alignment during the entire rolling treatment, as shown in the two photos in Figure 8-3. Maintaining proper alignment of the spine throughout the entire rolling treatment involves your head, neck, shoulder blades, core muscles, pelvis and, of course, the spine itself.

In Figure 8-3a you can see no excess rotation is allowed from the pelvis, the spine, the rib cage, the shoulders, the neck, and the head. Simply stated, the left side of the body is balanced with the right side of the body.

In Figure 8-3b you can see strong muscles and strong focus to maintain an aligned spine and body throughout the roller treatment. I encourage the use of a large wall mirror to reinforce a balanced body when rolling in a side position.

One last point regarding the importance of always maintaining an aligned spine when rolling any body part: By doing so, the roller treatments are much more effective, and your risk of injury is greatly reduced.

TIP

Here are some tips for keeping your spine in alignment as you roll:

>> **Keep your head on straight.** Look straight forward without twisting your spine. Imagine a straight line running through your nose, chin, sternum, and navel.

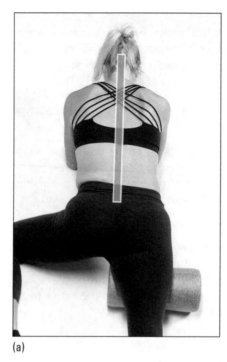 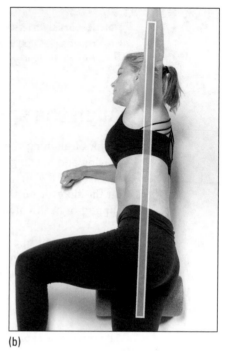

FIGURE 8-3:
A well-aligned
spine.

(a)

(b)

Photography by Haim Ariav & Klara Cu

>> **Maintain low back sway.** Maintain your natural standing position, using a low back curve, or "sway," when you're rolling.

>> **Keep breathing.** By *not* holding your breath, your diaphragm is more relaxed and your muscles are better fueled to do their jobs.

>> **Keep your chin over your ribs.** Your chin is the gatekeeper for the top half of your spine, so don't let it bail out forward. Keep your chin tucked backward so it's always resting directly above your ribs.

Breathe

Without proper breathing, the other rules are useless. As noted in the title of this chapter, "Working *With* Your Muscles, Not *Against* Them," your muscles' ability to return to being functional bone–movers is directly related to your ability to breathe slowly and deeply.

Imagine yourself rolling a sore muscle but holding your breath. When you do this, your blood pressure ramps up, your heart rate skyrockets, and the tension in the muscle quickly increases. With just those three physical responses instantly taking place, it's almost impossible for your muscle to relax.

REMEMBER

The take-home point: Rolling with improper breathing can make muscles tighter instead of looser.

TIP

To make sure you're breathing properly, inhale slowly, deeply, and loudly. Follow this with a relaxed, comfortable exhale.

PT NOTE

Were you surprised to see the word *loudly*? I emphasize that point to my patients because it's so important. Deliberately loud breathers are naturally deeper breathers. Loud breathing is also a great way to protect your private space. It lets everyone around you know you're locked in and focused.

Never. Stop. Breathing.

Slow your roll

Keep in mind that your objectives with roller treatments are to relax muscles, reduce pain, and increase body mobility.

REMEMBER

In order for the roller techniques I share with you in this book to work, you need a slow and consistent roller speed. This element of roller treatment allows your body the necessary time to make positive changes.

To better explain this point, I'll walk you through two examples, literally.

> **Scenario 1:** Imagine yourself walking down the sidewalk in your shiny new sneakers. You walk 300 yards to mail a letter, then another 300 yards back home. For the first leg of the trek, all is fine. No problems, no concerns. In the home-stretch, without warning, you step on a razor-sharp edge of the concrete, which stabs your right arch. Think of how your entire body responds to that sudden isolated pain. The sharp object is gone and you're not bleeding, but your arch, toes, ankle, knee, and hip have instantly changed. You probably limp all the way home, and most of your right leg muscles are now much tighter.

> **Scenario 2:** Imagine yourself taking the same walk as you did in Scenario 1. During that 600-yard jaunt, your right sock develops a small fold in the arch. It, too, does not feel good, but it's more an annoying pressure–type of discomfort. Compared to the sharp pain you felt in Scenario 1, this pain comes on *slowly* with less intensity. Here in Scenario 2, your brain, muscles, and joints have ample time to analyze and interpret the stimulus in your right arch. Your brain can clearly understand all the issues impacting your body. Without alarm, your brain, muscles, and joints quickly

synchronize their efforts to dissipate your body weight to a different part of the foot, arch, and toes to improve your symptoms.

That's a long explanation, but it's necessary to ensure you thoroughly appreciate this key rule for rolling slowly. When you *slowly* introduce roller pressure on muscle trigger points or adhesions, the body and brain have time to manage the stimulus in a positive, proactive way. By rolling *fast*, you're introducing the pain in a quick, insulting manner. The brain and body are forced to react in a protective, defensive manner.

Follow these tips to help ensure you roll slowly and smoothly.

>> Understand the starting and finishing points for your roller treatments, to be learned in Chapters 16 to 20.

>> Know the direction you will move on the roller or ball.

>> Start both the movement and the deep breathing in a slow, steady manner.

Seek and destroy trigger points

Trigger points, also known as *myofascial trigger points,* are localized, painful knots within and around skeletal muscles. They are hyperirritable, restrictive bands of tightness that can involve muscle, tendons, fascia, scar tissue, and skin. As shown in Figure 8-4, trigger points can cause surrounding soft tissue to be painful, restrictive, and limiting.

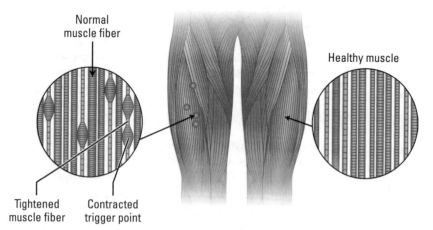

FIGURE 8-4: Our muscles' troublemaker: the myofascial trigger point.

©John Wiley & Sons, Inc.

OUCH

Trigger points hurt. They make your muscles and joints tighter. They make your muscles weaker. They slow you down. They are not your friends! I want to show you how to "seek and destroy" annoying trigger points so you can get back to living an active and healthy lifestyle. Seeking and destroying trigger points with a roller is fun and effective.

TIP

To seek and destroy your own trigger point, follow these steps:

1. **Breathe.**

   Remember — slow, deep, and loud.

2. **Seek.**

   Use the roller to find a tender trigger point. Let the roller get on top of the "painful grapes," as I call them.

3. **Melt.**

   Allow the roller to melt into the muscle while you take slow, deep breaths.

4. **Move.**

   Slowly move the joint above and/or below the roller, twice, from 45 to 90 degrees, remembering to breathe slowly, deeply, and loudly.

5. **Repeat.**

   Repeat the Breathe, Seek, Melt, Move sequence until all the painful myofascial trigger points have been treated. For most "Roller Rookies" new to this exciting new hobby, they will typically find three to five trigger points in each muscle group.

You may be wondering, "What's the outcome, the end result when I destroy my trigger points?" Great question. The answer: a more relaxed, limber, "loosey-goosey," responsive muscle. As you discover in Chapter 16 how to perfect the pre-roller test and post-roller test, within five minutes you'll be smiling at how much better your muscle will feel when your myofascial trigger points are tamed!

Move the muscle

Did I happen to mention that rollers can be uncomfortable? I thought so.

OUCH

Now that I've mentioned the pink, painful elephant in the room, it's time to tell you about another uncomfortable topic. My "fifth" of adding joint motion to your roller treatment will make the treatment more effective, but in doing so, it will also make it more painful.

I can hear you now: "This guy is supposed to be eliminating my pain, yet here he is telling me his fifth rule will make my roller treatments more painful!" Touché. Your point is a valid one. But I can explain why this last rule is a major game changer when it comes to decreasing your muscle pain and restoring your active pain-free lifestyle.

Our bodies are dynamic and motion-driven. Be it in sports or life, we move, we jump, we twist, we bend. To do this effectively, with no pain, we need our muscles to be responsive throughout their own large range of motion. So, if we only perform roller treatments to unlock our muscles in their resting positions, it does not guarantee those muscles and tendons will remain unlocked and mobile when they're stretched and loaded in other positions or postures.

Adding motion for Level 2 self-myofascial unlocking techniques is explained in greater detail in Chapters 16 to 20, based on the body part being treated.

When you add motion to a muscle that is being compressed and unlocked by a roller, the treatment range for that muscle is instantly expanded. Now the treated muscle, tendons, and fascia are stretched and reset throughout a larger range of motion. It's important to note that this is very different from simply stretching the muscle. During a roller treatment, the trigger points within the muscle and surrounding soft tissue are relaxed with the self-myofascial unlocking via the roller. Then the treated muscle is elongated. As demonstrated in Figure 8-5, this is another example of working *with* the muscle and surrounding soft tissue. Compare this treatment approach to just a passive stretch of the muscle and its trigger points, where the tight and painful muscle will most likely fight or resist the stretch.

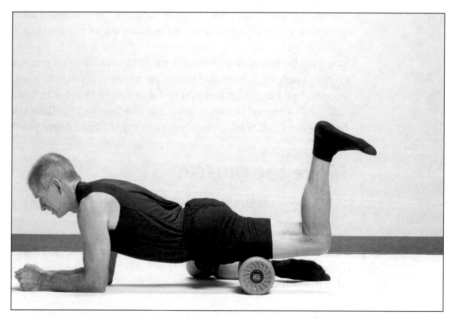

FIGURE 8-5:
An active contraction on one side of a body part helps the roller relax the muscle on the other side of the body part.

Photography by Haim Ariav & Klara Cu

There's one additional, exciting benefit to share regarding this new bonus rule: *reciprocal inhibition*. It sounds like a complicated exercise physiology term, but it's actually quite simple: Reciprocal inhibition is a neuromuscular reflex that relaxes the muscles on one side of a body part when the muscles on the opposite side of that body part are contracted (see Figure 8-6). It's similar to using a dimmer switch for your painful muscle!

The following table shows some examples of reciprocal inhibition.

When These Muscles Contract	These Muscles Relax
Biceps	Triceps
Wrist flexors (palm side)	Wrist extensors (backside)
Chest	Upper back
Shoulder internal rotators	Shoulder external rotators
Abs	Lower back
Quads	Hamstring
Glutes	Hip flexors
Ankle dorsi flexors (front of shins)	Calves (back of shins)

Consider the following example of how we can use reciprocal inhibition to treat a common injury. Let's assume you have chronic tennis elbow with overly tight and sore muscles on the top side of your forearm. I would use a small roller ball on the angry trigger points located throughout the five wrist extensor muscles on the top side of your forearm. I'd ask you to slowly flex your wrist, moving the palm-side of your hand upward towards the ceiling.

Stay with me for this key detail, as it will help you master this important technique. By contracting your wrist flexor muscles (located on the palm-side of your forearm), with the roller ball compressing a trigger point located in the muscle belly of a wrist extensor muscles (located on the back-side of your forearm), you are producing a reciprocal inhibition.

The reciprocal inhibition relaxes the muscles that are being stretched when the muscles on the opposite side of the body part are being contracted.

So, for this example, the tight and painful wrist extensors — which originate at the outside of the elbow where tennis elbow occurs — are quickly relaxed from both the unlocking technique from the roller and from the added benefit of a reciprocal inhibition.

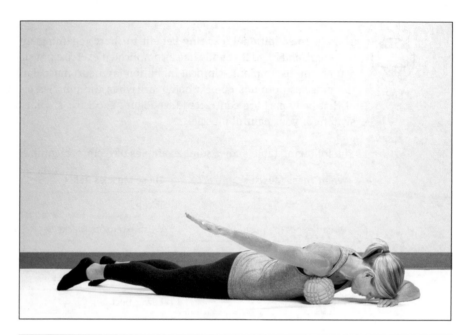

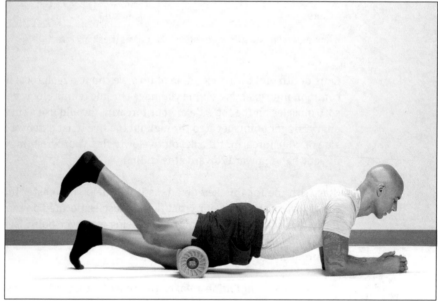

FIGURE 8-6:
Reciprocal
inhibition in
action.

Photography by Haim Ariav & Klara Cu

Working with Your Muscles by Keeping Them Hydrated

REMEMBER

If we want our bodies to function consistently and proficiently at a high level, we need to give them plenty of water. Water is not a fuel, per se, but the estimated 30 trillion cells in your body need water to do their job.

Following are the five main functions of water in the human body:

>> Cell life

>> Transport

>> Chemical reactions

>> Temperature regulation

>> Waste excretion

"Is water the only thing your muscles need to be hydrated?" you ask. No. To avoid turning this into a diet and nutrition book, I'll keep this topic simple. I've learned from working hands-on with thousands of athletes — from professional football players to Ironman triathletes to weekend warriors to Olympians to high school runners to stay-at-home mothers to PGA golfers — that keeping hydration simple works amazingly well for 80 percent of athletes. The remaining 20 percent may have an unusual gastrointestinal system or an altered nutritional need that requires an individualized nutritional plan. I'll assume that you fall into the 80-percent silo.

Your body needs these four items in this order:

>> Water

>> Sodium (salt)

>> Electrolytes

>> Calories

REMEMBER

Try this simplified hydration plan when exercising over 30 minutes, especially in a hot environment. As with any food or fluid you consume, always monitor how your body responds to ensure the plan works for you. If you have any medical conditions or nutritional complications, consult your physician for guidance.

During my 20 years as the Head Athletic Trainer/Physical Therapist for the Jacksonville Jaguars (from 1994 to 2014), keeping my players and staff safe in the brutal Florida heat and humidity was no easy task. My staff and I learned from both the experts and our athletes how to manage the hydration and nutrition of 90 professional football players wearing 25 pounds of equipment, exercising at a high intensity for up to five hours per day in the intense summer sun in the "Sunshine State."

To test my heat and hydration expertise, I took my skills and theories to the ultimate tests. I competed in the three hottest Ironman Triathlons in the world. Those three triathlons took place in Hawaii, Lanzarote in the Canary Islands, and Brazil. If you don't know what an Ironman Triathlon entails, the one-day event starts with a 2.4-mile swim, followed by a 112-mile bike race, and finally a 26.2-mile marathon run. I learned a great deal from those brutally hot and challenging events (see Figure 8-7). The lessons from those endeavors changed me as an athlete, as an athletic trainer and physical therapist, and as a heat and hydration mentor for athletes wanting to stay safe in extreme conditions.

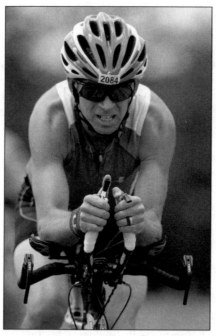

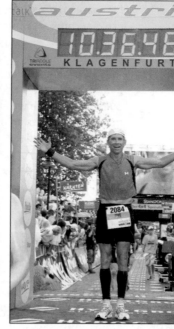

FIGURE 8-7: The author in Ironman Austria.

Photography by Haim Ariav & Klara Cu

My athletes embraced what we called the Ryan 50/50 Plan to stay properly hydrated. This plan provided them with the four key items (noted previously) your body needs to be safe and perform at an optimal level: water, sodium, electrolytes, and calories.

PT NOTE

The Ryan 50/50 Plan: 50 percent water/50 percent Gatorade before, during, and after practice. It's that simple.

To clarify,

>> Before the workout: 50 percent water/50 percent Gatorade

>> During the workout: 50 percent water/50 percent Gatorade

>> After the workout: 50 percent water/50 percent Gatorade

Good Roller Pain versus Bad Roller Pain

Not all pain is created equal. Think about the very worst physical pain you've ever experienced. Put yourself back into that uncomfortable place in time. Relive the intensity of that moment. Hear those sounds again: around you, in you, from you. Remember the very vivid images and thoughts that raced through your mind at shocking speeds. As you snap back to now, answer the following three questions:

Is your heart racing?

Are your palms sweaty?

Is your body having a hard time sitting still?

Even if the most painful moment of your life occurred 20-plus years ago, I bet the answer is *yes* to all three of these questions.

The painful experience you just relived is a perfect example of *bad pain*. Bad pain is often the result of working against our muscles and against our bodies. This is why even an isolated bad pain no bigger than the size of dime along, say, the joint-line of your knee negatively affects your entire body physically, emotionally, and even spiritually. With disheartening times like this we are often left with the troubling question: "*Is this bad pain working against my body, or is my entire body working against my bad pain?*"

I walked you through a painful time in your life not to make you uncomfortable, but to show you the wide range of pain we can experience as humans. We can learn a great deal about ourselves during times of bad pain. That intense and unnerving pain truly shows how we and those around us manage difficult times. Bad pain truly tests our toughness and fortitude.

Following are some examples of bad pain:

>> Nerve pain down the leg

>> Muscle tear

>> Blister on your foot

>> Muscle spasm

>> Torn muscle tendon

>> Broken bone

>> Ligament tear

>> Migraine headache

Meanwhile, there are many times in our lives when we experience a pain that enhances or helps us in some way. This is the type of pain we feel when a restricted or tight part of our body is treated and returns to its relaxed state. Oftentimes our body is compensating for a chronic injury or body imbalance. When we restore normal muscle function and joint range of motion with physical therapy techniques, it can be uncomfortable or painful. But compared to intense injury pain, this pain is obviously beneficial and ultimately rewarding.

This type of pain is what I refer to as *good pain*.

Unlike bad pain working against your body, good pain is the body's reaction when an activity or reaction is working with the body. Although lumped into the "pain" bucket, many of these symptoms can be viewed as a "feeling." Although these good pains can be uncomfortable, knowing they're accompanied by limited concern for negative outcomes or bodily harm makes them a welcome guest for an informed host.

To make a muscle stronger, the muscle fibers need to be overloaded and broken down. When the muscles fibers are repaired over the next 48 hours, they are stronger than they were originally. This process of overloading, breaking down, and regenerating is far from comfortable. But this is another example of a good pain. The deep muscle burn and fatigue with high-intensity, full range of motion exercise is a common example of a good pain being worth the final outcome of a stronger and longer muscle.

Following are some examples of good pain:

>> Muscle fatigue during exercise

>> Deep muscle massage

>> Releasing of scar tissue

>> Unlocking of a muscle/Releasing of a trigger point

>> Mild to moderate muscle stretch

>> Myofascial release

>> Relaxing a muscle spasm

REMEMBER

When you're rolling and you experience what I'll call *discomfort*, which sounds more inviting than *pain*, ask yourself the following question: "Is this a good pain or a bad pain?" If it's what you consider a bad pain, stop your rolling treatment immediately. But if you consider the discomfort a good pain, continue with your rolling treatment while also monitoring your symptoms.

PT NOTE

The last thing I want is for you to feel intense pain, just assuming that it's expected, and to blindly continue the treatment. Needless to say, this is a mistake that's likely to make your injury worse. I want you to keep the discomfort level of all your roller treatments and workouts mild to low-moderate. If you're experiencing any intense or shooting pain, stop the treatment/workout immediately.

exertion, be it work or play

» Learning how to accelerate your muscle recovery with a roller

» Avoiding common recovery mistakes

Chapter **9**

Supercharging Your Post-Workout Recovery with a Roller

When the work is done, it's time to relax and enjoy the fruits of our labor, right? Maybe it's after your record-setting run or that hard workout in the gym. Or maybe you just finished mowing the lawn or painting the house in the 95-degree heat.

Whatever it was that you did, your body deserves an active recovery. Notice that I said "active recovery," not "a cold beer and the couch." The latter will come later.

REMEMBER

Active recovery sessions don't need to be lengthy or complicated. The objective of these sessions is to accelerate the removal of waste products from your muscles, relax the soft tissue, and enhance the muscles' ability to take in good, healthy blood.

The Value of the Recovery

I think we can all agree: Cool-downs are not the most exciting part of our workouts. Few of us meet up with our friends after work to brag about how awesome our post-workout recoveries were last week. But if you truly want to stay active and pain-free, now is the time to sharpen your recovery skills with me. I will walk you through the steps to make your recovery game plan quick and effective.

PT NOTE

Being the physical therapy geek that I am, I like posting recovery and cool-down tips on my social media accounts. I make a strong effort to "stay in my lane." My professional "lane" or expertise involves the following five areas:

>> Sports medicine

>> Injury prevention

>> Injury management

>> Physical therapy

>> Active recovery

I'll let the many strong and highly skilled coaches and personal trainers out there teach you how to get faster and stronger. Those are not my strongest skill sets. My expertise is highly specialized in keeping you pain-free and, if you get injured, in helping you get back in the game quickly and safely.

Give Me Six: The Six-Minute Recovery Roll-Down

Let me teach you how to complete your recovery roll-down in a mere six minutes. This speed plan can be used to recover from a long workout, sitting at the desk, yard work, a car ride, uncomfortable dress shoes, a bad night of sleep, a long day on your feet, or just a stressful day.

Think of your recovery this way: accelerating your body's ability to get the *bad* stuff out of your muscles and the *good* stuff into your muscles.

Bad stuff you want to exit your muscles includes the following:

>> Lactate

>> Dead blood cells

- » Carbon dioxide
- » Hydrogen
- » Ethanol
- » Waste products
- » Heat

Good stuff you want to enter your muscles includes the following:

- » Oxygen
- » Water
- » Carbohydrates
- » Proteins
- » Fats
- » Calories
- » Electrolytes

Here is your six-minute recovery roll-down game plan. It will help you get the most from your hard work by reducing the risk of muscle tightness, joint stiffness, and overall soreness.

1. **90-second drink:** This is to replace what you just lost.

   Consume at least one 20-oz. bottle of 50-percent water and 50-percent electrolytes.

2. **2-minute drain:** Lie down and elevate your legs, as shown in Figure 9-1a.

   Allow gravity to aid in the removal of extremity waste products via your lymphatic and circulatory systems. During this time, wiggle your toes, pump your ankles as shown in Figure 9-1b, and bend your knees as shown in Figure 9-1c.

3. **30-second check:** Check your body for areas of tightness or pain, as shown in Figure 9-2.

   This is a quick and easy activity that includes marching in place, arm circles, squats, trunk twists, and toe touches.

4. **2-minute roll:** Seek and destroy any trigger points and trouble spots.

   Now that you know your trouble spots, perform a quick roll of those body parts (found in Chapters 16 to 20).

Grand total: 6 minutes

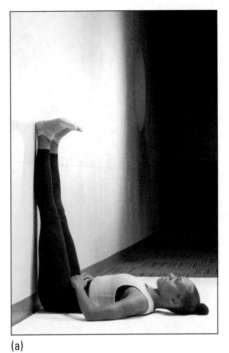

(a)

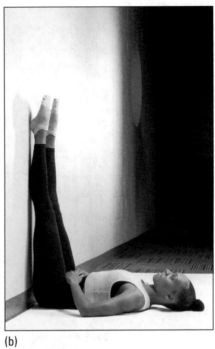

(b)

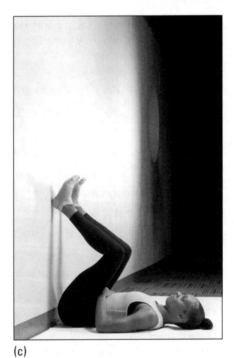

(c)

FIGURE 9-1:
Draining
the legs to
supercharge
your recovery.

Photography by Haim Ariav & Klara Cu

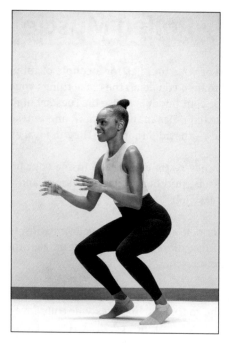

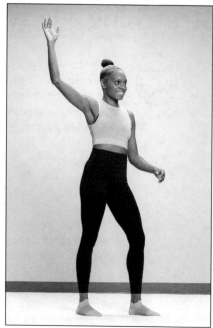

FIGURE 9-2: Squats and arm circles to assess what parts of your body need some rollin'.

Photography by Haim Ariav & Klara Cu

Those six minutes may have saved you days of discomfort, extremity stiffness, and limited joint range of motion. And if such a recovery is not performed, other body parts such as your lower back or knee may have become sore and concerning.

TIP

Instead, the new wiser-and-healthier you is pain-free, not taking anti-inflammatory medication, not Googling for cheap, pain-reducing remedies, and living a healthier, active lifestyle! That six minutes was truly "time well spent."

Injury prevention is not sexy, but it works. If you trust me to help you prevent injuries, in doing so, I will save you three things:

>> Time

>> Money

>> Pain

In our busy lives, those three things are extremely important to all of us.

Stretching a Freshly Rolled Muscle

PT NOTE

Put yourself in the place of your muscles for a couple of minutes. Your muscles have been working hard to help you do all the crazy things you do. Carrying those four boxes up the stairs at your buddy's house on Tuesday night — they did that. Walking what seemed like ten miles in the hot, new, and too-small dress shoes at the wedding last weekend — they did that, too. They're loyal and they work hard.

To make matters worse, they're tightly packed inside your body with countless other muscles, blood vessels, nerves, lymphatic vessels, and all the other stuff. Being a muscle is not an easy job.

When the hard work is done, it's time to show your muscles, tendons, and fascia some love. After completing a short roller treatment on your muscles, it's time to reward them with an easy stretch.

And I have to tell you, the more you do this quick combination of post-workout rolling and stretching, the more your muscles will truly love it! Let me explain why. Muscles can only pull, they cannot push. So, they're constantly compressing themselves to help you move, lift, twist, and pull. Following any hard work, your muscles and the tight, fibrous fascia around them end up restricted and tight. Using a roller after any exertion keeps the soft tissue (muscle, tendons, fascia, blood vessels, lymphatic vessels, and skin) loose and limber, while the busy recovery process takes place.

REMEMBER

My roller-then-stretching plan steamrolls and then lengthens the soft tissue, as all the bad stuff leaves the area and the good stuff effortlessly flows in.

Now, with the muscle group freshly rolled after your workout, stretching the muscle helps to restore the muscle and fascia back to its normal resting length.

PT NOTE

An added bonus to stretching a muscle that has been freshly rolled is how it can protect the muscle's tendons. Tendons attach the muscles to the bone. By stretching a more-relaxed muscle, thanks to the roller, you can apply a more effective stretch to the tendons at either end of the muscle.

TIP

As a quick reference guide to help you incorporate stretching into your daily routine, here are the typical muscle groups requiring consistent stretching.

>> Upper body

- Chest muscles

- Latissimus dorsi (lats)

- » Lower body
  - Quadriceps muscles
  - Hamstring muscles
- » Core/spine
  - Hip flexors
  - Sides of neck/upper trapezius muscles

For more details and direction, check out Chapter 21. It's packed with roller workouts and stretches for your three body zones: upper body, lower body, and core/spine. Spend some time learning the easy-to-learn-but-challenging-to-complete exercises related to your body part(s) in need of extra care.

Common Recovery Mistakes to Avoid

Following are some mistakes you want to avoid making when it comes to recovery:

- » Not hydrating properly with water and electrolytes
- » Consuming "energy drinks" instead of electrolyte-based fluids
- » Skipping a cool-down, roller treatment, stretching, or low-intensity movements
- » Stretching too aggressively
- » Immediate inactivity, aka "just chillin'"
- » Not consuming healthy calories within a 45-minute window post-workout
- » Delaying body-core cooling when exercising in a hot environment

3

Meeting the Muscles You're Rolling Over, and More

Chapter **10**

Discovering What's Under the Skin: Knowing Your Anatomy

'm very grateful to have spent the past 35 years in the sports medicine field. During that time, I've witnessed firsthand how the healthiest athletes are the ones who better understanding and appreciation of their bodies. The healthier athletes aren't doctors, but they do understand how their body maintenance habits influence how they move. Healthier athletes also spend the time to become students of their bodies, learning which rollers, strengthening exercises, stretches, hydration plans, and foods help them manage their pain.

PT NOTE

I am excited to share sports medicine secrets and tricks typically reserved for world-class athletes with individuals like you looking for healthy ways to stay pain-free without medication. It's my passion to share these elite sports medicine secrets with non-professional athletes just like you. My professional mission statement: *To enhance the health of others.*

In this chapter, I take you on an adventurous ride under our body's largest organ: the skin. Most of the body structures covered in this chapter will be somewhat familiar to you. Anatomical structures like muscles, tendon, bones, joints, and fascia are probably somewhat familiar, but it's the skills and functions of these body parts which I hope will fascinate you.

This chapter serves as an anatomy appetizer, if you will. You get the basics on the important orthopedic or skeletal stuff under the skin, which helps you walk, bend, twist, squat, lift, jump, and more. (In Part 3, I go deeper into these body parts before I show you how to treat your tight and painful muscles and fascia in Part 4.)

Muscles and Tendons

Muscles are the machines that move your bones. Muscles help you maintain your posture and your balance. Muscles are a collection of thousands of small muscle fibers, as shown in Figure 10-1. I won't bore you with a heavy anatomy lesson describing the sliding filament theory on muscle contractions. Keeping it simple, each skeletal muscle is a collection of thousands of tiny muscle fibers, all neatly wrapped together by, you guessed it, fascia. Each of the 600-plus muscles in the human body has its own unique shape, angle, attachments, length, contraction capacity, and arrangement of fibers, based on its function.

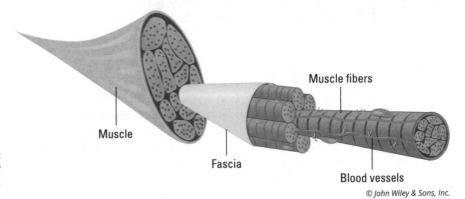

Muscle fibers

Muscle

Fascia

Blood vessels

© John Wiley & Sons, Inc.

FIGURE 10-1:
The anatomy
of a muscle.

Tendons, located at both ends of a muscle, attach muscles to bones. While muscles are able to contract and stretch, tendons are tight and dense. Muscles are more like thick rubber bands, and tendons are more like leather belts attached to both ends of the stretchy muscles. When a muscle contracts, it pulls on its tendon(s) anchored to a bone. The force of the muscle contraction travels through the muscle, then through the tendon to the bone. If the force of the muscle contraction is stronger than the resistance of the bone and the object attached to that bone, the bone will move.

A muscle can generate three types of muscle contractions:

>> **Concentric contraction.** The working muscle generates a force that is greater than the external load, allowing the muscle to shorten.

For example, your arm biceps muscle bends your elbow, which raises your hand towards your shoulder.

>> **Eccentric contraction.** The working muscle generates a force that is less than the external load, forcing the muscle to lengthen. In the fitness world, this type of contraction is referred to as a "negative" contraction.

For example, your arm biceps muscle slowly allows the arm to straighten at your elbow, which lowers your hand towards the floor.

>> **Isometric contraction.** The working muscle generates a force that is equal to the external load, resulting in no change in muscle length or joint angle.

For example, when your arm biceps muscle contracts with the same force as your triceps muscle, this results in no elbow motion. This is the type of contraction someone makes when they strike a "strongman pose" to show how big their arm muscles are.

REMEMBER

Understanding the three types of contractions will help you to move better with a lower risk of injury. Let me explain: When performing a familiar movement, your body knows how it wants to function. Whether bending down to tie your shoes, running down the street, or throwing a baseball, your body's muscles, tendons, fascia, and joints have a plan. But when any of the involved muscles are locked down because of a trigger point, overly tight fascia, or weakness, your body immediately switches to Plan B. In most cases, Plan B is not doing you any favors other than just trying to accomplish your end goal (tie the shoe, run, throw the ball). With Plan B, the sequence and type of muscle contracts is now altered. This puts unnecessary stress on soft tissue that may not be properly prepared for the workload. This is the "perfect storm" for an overuse injury. Rollers are effective in restoring muscle, tendon, fascia, and joint mobility so the treated muscles have the unrestricted ability to generate all three types of contractions.

Bones and Joints

Your 206 bones are the building blocks of your body keeping you upright and mobile. Without bones, you'd resemble a jellyfish. Bones give you size while protecting your precious cargo, including your brain, heart, lungs, and kidneys.

Joints, on the other hand, enable you to move your bones with great precision. Joints are like the hinges on a door, and their intricate positions, angles, and surface areas dictate the direction and range of your movements. Some joints, like your shoulders and upper spine, allow for a large range of motion, while other joints, like your hip and lower spine, are more restricted by their joint surfaces and therefore allow for a more restricted range of motion.

OUCH

If you are older or have previous joint injuries, you may be suffering from joint arthritis. Arthritis is a loss of articular cartilage at the end of the bones that form the two sides of a joint. The damage to the joint surface typically results in a progressive reduction in the range of motion of the joint. This is why it's extremely important for an arthritic joint to maintain its range of motion to preserve the health and function of the joint.

WARNING

If a hinge on an old door becomes rusty, the last thing you should do is stop moving the door. If you limit the movement of the door, the hinge becomes increasingly stiff. The same is true with an arthritic joint. Having a safe and healthy plan to maintain a maximum joint range of motion needs to be a top priority for all of us at any age. Inactivity and limiting motion of an arthritic joint is the perfect game plan for a stiff and painful joint. That's a bad game plan! Think about elderly people in your life who struggle to move. Most of them struggle because their joints are not healthy.

Now you have a tool (rollers) and a game plan (this book) to preserve your joints and the muscles that move those joints! When you use a roller, you enhance the health of the muscles and fascia above and below a joint to significantly reduce the stress on the joint. By increasing the blood flow, flexibility, and lymphatic drainage for soft tissue, you help ensure the surrounding joints can move with less effort.

Fascia

In my opinion, fascia is the most underappreciated tissue in the human body. Also referred to as *myofascial tissue* because of its close intertwining with muscle tissue, fascia is a thin yet very strong fibrous connective tissue (you can refer to Chapter 6 for a very cool image of fascia). It's found throughout your body, and surrounds every muscle, organ, bone, blood vessel, lymphatic vessel, and nerve in your body. Think of it as a giant spiderweb that spreads from your toes to your head.

It may be thin and filled with many holes, but fascia is very strong. Much like muscle, fascia is able to contract and restrict joint motion, and be a source of pain.

Fascia is categorized as a connective tissue. It may not be solid like bone, but never underestimate the strength of fascia and its impact on the function of your body. The functional impact on the muscles of your body can be good or bad. If the fascia is properly aligned and mobile, like a well-fitted pair of leg tights you'd wear to the gym, it helps the muscles and joints to be responsive and powerful. But if your fascia is bound down and restrictive like a wet pair of tight jeans, it makes your muscles and joints weak and stiff.

I'm assuming the last few paragraphs have opened your eyes to the amazing world of fascia. I often use the following analogy with my patients:

> Fascia is to the human body what sand is to the beach. When we're having fun at the beach, we rarely focus on the sand or sing sand's praises. But without it, the beach would suck!

I get excited about fascia for many reasons. When athletes think of speed, flexibility, and power, most of them don't think about their fascia. That's a mistake. Fascia plays a crucial role in supporting muscles and the strength those muscles generate. Meanwhile, fascia is too often a source of diffuse and difficult-to-diagnose pain. You may not be as excited about fascia as I am — yet — but I bet your eyes have been opened to this mysterious tissue that's constantly altering your posture, muscle flexibility, joint range of motion, and body pain. (To find out even more about fascia and how it impacts your body, check out Chapter 13.)

With all this being said, the take-home point I want you to remember is as follows: "My fascia is very important and I will learn how to keep my fascia happy." Just like an unmanaged ivy vine growing wild in the woods, unmanaged fascia can quickly get out of control and wreak havoc on your entire body. Unmanaged fascia *will* bind down your muscles, restrict your joints, and produce chronic pain. You don't want that! Meanwhile, rollers are a great tool to keep your fascia happy.

What's a Myofascial Trigger Point?

Even for medical experts, defining a trigger point is not as simple as it sounds. The wide range of definitions and tissue sources for painful trigger points makes defining a trigger point confusing for all of us. There are many in the orthopedic world who claim trigger points don't even exist. But for those of us who have suffered from painful trigger points, forgetting them is impossible.

According to the website Physio-pedia.com, a trigger point is defined as "a hyper-irritable spot, a palpable nodule in the taut bands of a skeletal muscle's fascia."

You'll see the use of two titles, *trigger points* and *myofascial trigger points*, throughout this book. For the purpose of this book for treating muscle ailments, the two terms can be used interchangeably. Knots, localized hyperactivities, and trigger points within a muscle typically involve both muscle and fascial tissue.

Because of the trigger point's localized spot of hyperactivity in the muscle and fascia, the function of the entire muscle altered. Even if the location of this trigger point is isolated to a very small point in a single muscle, the trigger point can alter the function of the many surrounding muscles, causing pain and body compensation. Think how quickly a small, painful "knot" in your calf muscle spirals into a tight hamstring, stiff knee, tight lower back, noticeable limp, and bad attitude.

OUCH

And when it comes to anyone who is active, trigger point pain forces them to compensate in the way they move, which typically results in more pain and compensation, as shown in Figure 10-2. Needless to say, the downward cycle of trigger point pain, which leads to stiffness, then to abnormal movement, and then to more pain, is a bad thing.

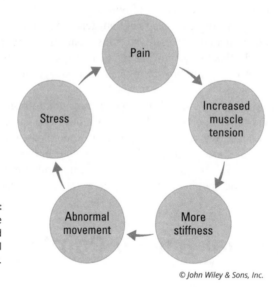

FIGURE 10-2: The cycle of pain and abnormal movement.

© John Wiley & Sons, Inc.

Types of trigger points are as follows:

>> **Active trigger point.** An extremely tender knot located within your myofascial tissue.

>> **Latent trigger point.** A palpable localized knot that is dormant or inactive. This point becomes active with trauma or stress.

>> **Secondary trigger point.** A mildly tender nodule that becomes active with the presence of an active trigger point in another muscle.

>> **Satellite myofascial trigger point.** A tender area activated by the presence of a nearby painful trigger point.

I love the famous quote, "The best defense is a good offense," for many reasons. The athlete in me has seen the same mindset play out well in sports as well as the military. The physical therapist and athletic trainer in me loves to tweak this quote to help keep my patients injury-free.

I'll put a sports medicine spin on this quote, as follows: "The best injury prevention (defense) is an aggressive body maintenance routine (offense)."

>> **Defense:** I think injury prevention works because it is a defensive approach to keep you out of danger or from getting hurt. To prevent the trauma of the ball or opponent from hurting you, you automatically take a defensive posture or position.

>> **Offense:** An aggressive maintenance routine is proactive. You study your opponents and develop a game plan to prepare your skills and abilities to attack when necessary. It's clearly an offensive approach to prepare your body for battle.

Enough with my novice approach to philosophical literature. I can hear you now: *"Get back in your sports medicine lane, Mike!"* Touché. Sorry. Where were we? Oh yes, trigger points.

The best way to manage trigger points is to avoid getting trigger points. This is another good example of the quote, "Prevention is the best form of medicine." And the best way to avoid trigger points is to manage the mobility of your muscles and fascia. That is not always an easy thing to do.

The Treasure Hunt

Because fascia travels in multiple directions with no specific beginning or end, restrictions and adhesions in fascia can be difficult to find. As a physical therapist, I use trigger points like valuable clues on a fun anatomical treasure hunt.

As a person seeking ways to move better with less pain, your treasure hunt is valuable. Your ability to find your source of pain or restriction will save you valuable time (less wasted time in a doctor's office and explaining your injury to others) and valuable money (unnecessary medical tests, appointments, and medicine).

Empowered with your new treasure hunt mindset, you will love Chapter 22. I share with you my secret injury evaluator formula fine-tuned from 26 years in the National Football League rehabilitating professional football players.

Let's get back to the treasure hunt, shall we?

The clues (painful trigger points) on the treasure map (the body) help me find hidden treasures (bound-down fascia). I use my special treasure tools (fingers, elbows, heels, and rollers) to dig up (release) the fascia and muscles. Lastly, I simply return to the clue (painful trigger point) to see if the pain is gone or significantly reduced.

A body treasure hunt analogy may sound corny to you, and you're probably right. It's true: I'm a bit strange when it comes to helping non-professional athletes to stay healthy and active. But that's fine with me because I want — no, I *need* — my clients to understand their anatomy and my game plans to keep them healthy. I don't mind if they look at me funny or think of me as "odd," as long as they truly understand, remember, and benefit from my sports medicine information. My business motto is as follows:

> Provide sports medicine information and treatment that is *easy* to understand, *simple* to apply, and produces *fast results.*

If my wellness information accomplishes those three goals, then my clients win and I'm happy. A win-win.

Did you notice that I added a little change to the treatment game plan? Instead of simply treating the trigger points, we are also looking for and treating areas of restrictions and tightness. This is helpful because a trigger point can be influenced by tight muscles, fascia, and skin many inches away from the trigger point. So, you are using a roller to treat not only the painful trigger point, but also areas of simple tightness and pressure above and below the trigger point.

Here are some signs and symptoms of trigger point and myofascial restrictions:

>> Deep localized pain

>> Palpable firmness/knot

>> Dull ache

>> Numbness

>> Generalized pressure and tightness

>> Tingling

>> Muscle tightness/cramp

>> Muscle fatigue

>> Referred or diffuse pain

Those symptoms are wide ranging. The key trait of a myofascial trigger point and fascia restriction is the localized nature of the symptoms with no specific trauma related to the injury. Other injuries or pathologies may have similar signs but also variations in their causes and symptoms. Table 10-1 shows some examples of differentiating between sources of muscle pain.

TABLE 10-1   ## Sources of Muscle Pain

Diagnosis	Cause	Symptoms
Myofascial trigger point (TrP)	Poor posture	Localized taut plus painful nodule
	Muscle imbalance	Referred pain with pressure
	Tight fascia	Localized muscle fatigue
Muscle strain	Trauma	Immediate localized pain
		Swelling, bleeding
		Increased pain with muscle contraction
Fibromyalgia	Infection	Widespread pain
	Genetics	Total body fatigue

REMEMBER

This treasure hunt game is a helpful treatment plan that you can also use. It gives you a game plan to improve your mobility and reduce your pain. I play this treatment game with both my physical therapy patients and myself.

TIP

A key tip for reducing the restrictive traits of fascia and myofascial trigger points is to find and treat them early. The earlier you find the trigger points and the restrictions, the easier they are to treat and eliminate.

Think back to the times when you had painful knots or general tightness in your muscles: the "kink" in your neck you woke up with after falling asleep on the couch while watching a long movie; the painful knot in your hamstring after four hours of paperwork; or the tight calf you suffered with last week, thanks to the new sweet-looking shoes you just bought.

The sooner you treated those ailments, the more quickly they disappeared and the better you felt. The hot shower and self-massage on the neck kink did the trick. Looking over that shoulder while driving the car 45 minutes later was not a problem. But that tight calf, the one you just ignored and hoped would simply disappear, was a whole different story. You just limped around the office showing off your pretty new shoes, thinking, "Yeh, this calf will take care of itself. It'll be fine tomorrow." Three days later, your calf, hamstring, and lower back were tight and painful.

Early intervention is important if you want your muscles and joints to stay happy. If your car needs a wheel alignment because of only one poorly positioned wheel, the longer you drive the misaligned car, the more stress you put on the car's brakes, struts, steering, and tires. Performing a simple and inexpensive wheel alignment for that one wheel saves complicated and expensive repairs down the road.

Your body responds in a similar manner. Fixing your minor ailments early will keep your muscles and joints happy *and* help you avoid painful and slow healing injuries down the road.

Chapter **11**
Upgrading Your Posture

"Sit up straight."

"Pull those shoulders back."

"Stop slumping in your chair."

Do those quotes bring you back to your childhood like they do for me? I was the youngest of five children. During our younger years, we were always reminded to practice strong posture. Unfortunately, many of us, myself included, don't always heed that wise posture advice in our later years.

In this chapter, I cover the importance of good posture and how posture impacts your life. To make it easy for you to improve your posture, I've broken down the key body parts that make your posture good or bad. With today's smartphones, you can quickly take photos of yourself to compare your body positions to the "perfect posture" and "poor posture" photos in this chapter.

Why Good Posture Is So Important

During your early years when your body is growing, proper posture is crucial because your body posture can influence the manner in which your bones grow. Your growth plates are the location close to the ends of your long bones where bone growth takes place. The cartilage plates close or calcify near the end of puberty.

For girls this typically takes place between the ages of 13 to 15, while boys tend to bloom later, so their growth plates close between the approximate ages of 15 to 17.

PT NOTE

So, if our bones stopped growing decades ago, why is it important for us as adults to worry about our posture? There are many reasons, some of which are in the following list. A simple way to look at why adult posture is so important relates to how our bodies function. Proper posture (Figure 11-1) helps the body function better with less effort. Poor posture (Figure 11-2) makes your body work harder, forcing the muscles to struggle in pain. It's that simple.

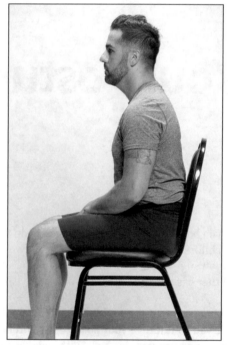

Photography by Haim Ariav & Klara Cu

FIGURE 11-1:
Strong sitting posture.

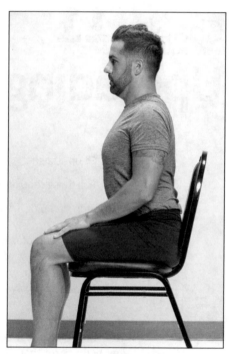

Photography by Haim Ariav & Klara Cu

FIGURE 11-2:
Poor sitting posture.

REMEMBER

Following are some benefits of strong posture:

>> Reduced pressure on the spine

>> Less effort to move

>> Fewer headaches

>> Less lower back pain

- » More energy
- » Improved workouts
- » Improved sleep
- » Reduced joint stress
- » Improved active movements
- » Reduced pressure on spinal nerves exiting and entering the spine
- » Increased height
- » More room for your organs to work their magic
- » Improved self-esteem and confidence

Understanding Posture

Okay, so we can all agree that posture is important for our body and our mind. We can look at someone and see if, generally speaking, they have good or bad posture. But evaluating our own posture is not so easy.

One of the reasons why understanding our own postural needs is so difficult is our poor understanding of our spine and torso muscles. It doesn't help that those muscles are hidden behind us, completely out of our view.

PT NOTE

You have dozens of smaller stabilizing muscles associated with your spine, positioned between your pelvis and skull. Each of those strong skeletal muscles has important roles related to posture and movement. Well-conditioned postural muscles tend to possess great endurance. They have the ability to hold spinal structures like the skull, neck, rib cage, arms, shoulder blades, and pelvis in the same positions for hours. That's no easy task. But having the ability to do their job for long periods of time while you walk, twist, lift, and jump makes their skillsets even more impressive.

When it comes to proper posture involving the shoulders, controlling the position of the shoulder blades is key. Each shoulder blade has 17 muscles attached to it. Many of those specialized muscles have the responsibility of keeping the shoulder blades, which are the bases of both arms, in a very specific position in relationship to the spine and rib cage. Conversely, the smaller of the two pectoralis muscles on the front of the chest attaches to the front of the shoulder blade. *Teaser alert:* Unlocking the pectoralis minor muscle will be a high priority when treating your shoulders and improving your posture.

When improving posture, it's imperative that you both relax and lengthen the muscles on the front of the chest while you strengthen and shorten the muscles on the back of the chest.

Improving both shoulder posture and shoulder function is achieved with a simple game plan: Getting *longer* in the front of the shoulder and *stronger* in the back of the shoulder.

After years of poor posture, many of those smaller stabilizing muscles between your shoulder blades become too long and too weak. Meanwhile, other dominant chest and shoulder muscles become too short and strong. Reversing that muscle imbalance will be a core focus for you with your shoulder treatments.

With this chronic muscle imbalance involving the torso and spine, improving posture isn't as simple as our mothers made it sound. (No offense, Mom.) With your chest, upper back, and shoulder muscles naturally strong and inflexible, correcting your posture is more difficult than simply pulling your shoulders back. If you truly want better shoulder posture, you have to lengthen the muscles on the front side of the shoulders and chest while you strengthen and shorten the muscles between your shoulder blades.

If you're a camping enthusiast, you can think of fixing your posture just like you would fix an old-school tent with a leaning center pole (see Figure 11-3). To get the tent pole to return to its proper vertical position, you have to *lengthen* the ropes on one side of the tent and *shorten* the ropes on the opposite side of the tent. If you only fix one side the tent, there is no way the supporting pole can have "perfect posture" and do its job.

FIGURE 11-3:
Improving your spine posture is similar to improving the position of the center pole in a tent.

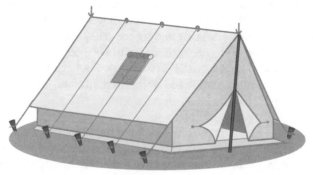

©John Wiley & Sons, Inc.

Key Landmarks for Evaluating Posture

I want to give you simple body landmarks and tips to help you evaluate your own posture. Before I do, I want you to look at how people around you sit, stand, and walk. Look around the room. Watch people on TV. Watch people young and old in your neighborhood. When you watch how everyone positions their body to do what they do, you'll probably come to the conclusion that everybody is truly different. Each of us has our own style of sitting, standing, and walking.

But within everyone's individual body styles is a basic "scaffolding" of bones and muscles. Each of us functions better when our scaffolding is properly positioned. When our body alignment is off, it weakens our body and forces us to work harder each and every day. How comfortable would you be climbing on a tall, leaning, rickety scaffolding? The same holds true for your muscles when your spine is leaning and unstable. With an imbalance and poor posture, the strong, dynamic muscles of your spine and torso are forced to struggle just to control your posture.

This section covers individual body parts. These body parts all stack on top of each other from your feet to your head. Much like children's building blocks stacked high, if you move one block, it will certainly affect every block above it.

TIP

If you're not clear on what you need to do to improve your posture, Part 4 in this book is packed with muscle treatments to help you lengthen tight and sore muscles that negatively impacting your posture. And when your posture is perfect, as we both know it will be, Chapter 21 will show you the perfect workouts and stretches to help you maintain your new strong and confident physique.

Head

Sign of poor posture: Your head is too far forward.

If the front of your chin is aligned in *front* of the ribs, then your head is too far forward. Notice I said "ribs" and not "chest." The landmark for your chin is the bony ribs, and not the pectoral muscles or chest (see Figure 11-4).

Sign of perfect posture: Your head is comfortably positioned over your upper ribs.

If a plumb bob or weighted line is dropped from the front of your chin, it should be aligned over the upper ribs, not in *front* of the ribs (see Figure 11-5).

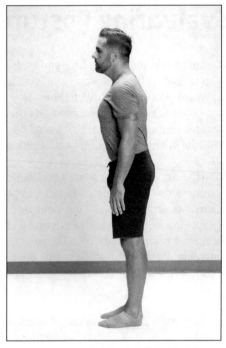

Photography by Haim Ariav & Klara Cu

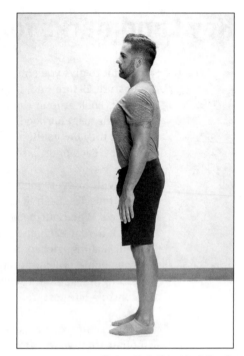

Photography by Haim Ariav & Klara Cu

FIGURE 11-4:
Poor head posture.

FIGURE 11-5:
Perfect head posture.

Shoulders

Sign of poor posture: Rounded shoulders with elevated shoulder blades.

With your back against a wall, the back of both shoulder *joints* should be touching the wall. If only the shoulder *blades* are touching the wall and the front of the shoulder joints are rolled forward, the shoulders are rounded and your posture is poor (see Figure 11-6).

Sign of perfect posture: Shoulder joints and shoulder blades are comfortably positioned back and downward towards the mid-spine.

With your back against a wall, the back of both shoulder joints will be touching the wall. And, ideally, the inside ridges of the two shoulder blades will be less than four inches apart (see Figure 11-7).

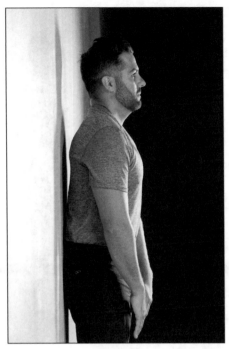

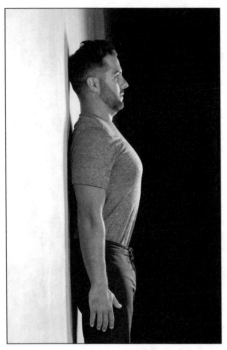

Photography by Haim Ariav & Klara Cu

Photography by Haim Ariav & Klara Cu

FIGURE 11-6:
Poor shoulder posture.

FIGURE 11-7:
Perfect shoulder posture.

Lower back

Sign of poor posture: Either exaggerated or no lordotic curve or "sway back." This may be accompanied by weak abdominal muscles.

Accurate lower back posture is best assessed with X-rays. With a clinical evaluation, the amount of the lower spine curve can be observed by viewing it from the side. The lack of any curve, seen as a straight spine, is typically more concerning than an exaggerated or excessive lumbar curve. A key finding for someone with a potentially troublesome exaggerated sway back is when the curve significantly increases with simple walking (see Figure 11-8).

Sign of perfect posture: Mild to moderate lordotic curve ("sway back") with strong, stabilizing abdominal muscles.

Perfect posture of the lower back equals strong abdominal muscles, strong lumbar muscles, a level pelvis, and flexible hamstrings. With walking, twisting, and high squats, the relationship between the lumbar curve and pelvis remains relatively consistent (see Figure 11-9).

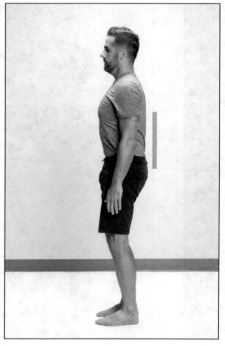

Photography by Haim Ariav & Klara Cu

FIGURE 11-8:
Poor lower back posture.

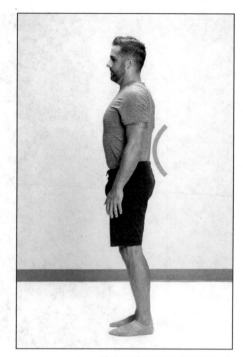

Photography by Haim Ariav & Klara Cu

FIGURE 11-9:
Perfect lower back posture

Pelvis

Sign of poor posture: Overly rotated forward with a lowered front of the pelvis.

An overly anteriorly rotated pelvis when standing is a common sign of someone with poor pelvis posture. This is usually accompanied by overly tight hip flexors and weak lower abdominal muscles (see Figure 11-10).

Sign of perfect posture: A level pelvis.

The position of the pelvis can vary, depending on many factors. A simple observation of a level pelvis can be done with you resting both hands on the upper ridge of your pelvis. Think of how an angry sports coach would stand on the sidelines. Generally speaking, the coach's index finger and thumb would be level with the floor. With a level pelvis, hopefully you also find the lower front half of your pelvis is pulled upward towards your navel (see Figure 11-11).

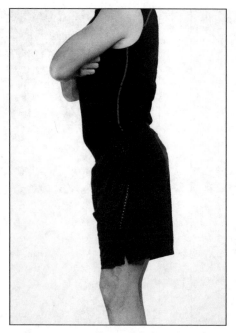

Photography by Haim Ariav & Klara Cu

FIGURE 11-10:
Poor pelvis posture.

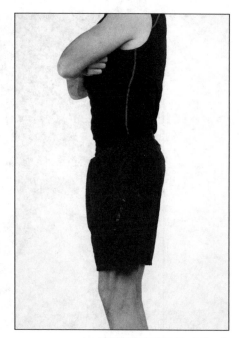

Photography by Haim Ariav & Klara Cu

FIGURE 11-11:
Perfect pelvis posture.

Feet

Sign of poor posture: Hyper-pronated with arches rolled inward.

Your feet function as your base of support, so a well-aligned base is vital for you to be active and pain-free. It's important for you to have some pronation when you walk and run, but too much pronation is a problem. Poor foot posture with excessive pronation is easy to spot. Stand barefoot with your feet parallel and shoulder-width apart. If your arches and heel bones cave inward as if the "balls" of the big toes are resting in a hole, excessive pronation is probably a problem. With moderate to severe hyper-pronation, you may also observe that your knees are leaning or angling inward (see Figure 11-12).

Sign of perfect posture: Moderate arches, vertical heel bone, and straight toes.

Perfect foot posture means your toes, feet, and ankle bones are pain-free, bilaterally symmetrical, and mobile. In addition, your heel bone appears to be completely vertical and the arches aren't too high or too low (see Figure 11-13).

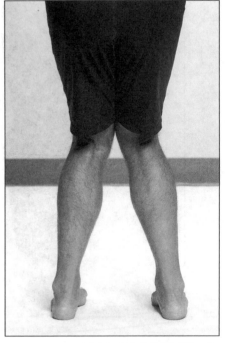
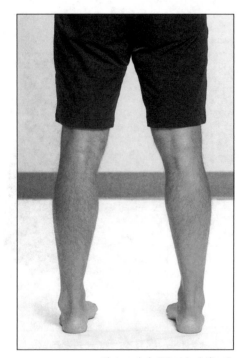

Photography by Haim Ariav & Klara Cux   *Photography by Haim Ariav & Klara Cu*

FIGURE 11-12:
Poor foot posture.

FIGURE 11-13:
Perfect foot posture.

What Does Perfect Posture Look Like?

PT NOTE

I'm a big fan of reverse engineering with my physical therapy patients. This is the process of thinking with the *end* in mind. The way I look at it, physical therapy reverse engineering is the mindset of putting yourself in a position of perfect body mechanics and health. Then, you start working backwards to determine the specific steps needed to reach your ideal final destination.

Put yourself in the position of having perfect posture. This is a great way to visualize what you need to achieve to end up with a balanced and pain-free body. As noted earlier, perfect posture just makes your life much easier. It takes less effort to maintain your balance, you easily move from point A to B, and the risk of an injury is dramatically reduced. How wonderful does that sound?

Perfect standing posture

I like to put my patients into a first-person perspective because it's a very powerful learning tool for both the body and mind. A first-person perspective put the person into the desired role and allowing them to see everything from an "inside" point of view. Unlike a second-person perspective when you watch someone else do something, as we do when we watch a movie or a sporting event.

For the following examples, I want you to see, feel, embrace and adapt to perfect standing posture:

» Your eyes are level with the floor.

» Your chin is comfortably positioned over the ribs.

» Your shoulders are drawn back and down with little effort.

» Your chest is strong and forward in a position of power.

» Your arms rest beside your hips, hanging naturally from well-positioned shoulders.

» The front of your pelvis is pulled upward with strong lower abdominal muscles and flexible hip flexors.

» Your knees are slightly bent with strong, engaged quad muscles.

» Your feet are strong and supportive with or without shoes.

Perfect sitting posture

As noted in the perfect standing posture introduction, this exercise will put you into a first-person point of view. In doing so, you will gain a powerful learning opportunity to help you quickly improve your sitting posture.

For the following examples, I want you to see, feel, embrace and adapt to perfect sitting posture:

» Your eyes are level with the floor.

» Your chin is comfortably positioned over the ribs.

» Your shoulders are drawn back and down.

» Your chest is strong and forward in a position of power.

» Your spine is only lightly touching the back of the chair because your back and core muscles, not the chair, are supporting your spine.

>> Your hands rest on your lap without pulling your elbows or shoulders forward.

>> Your pelvis is comfortably rolled forward to maintain the natural sway curve of your lower back.

>> Your knees are bent at approximately 90 degrees while your quads, hamstrings, and calves are relaxed, as your feet rest comfortably flat on the floor.

What Does Poor Posture Feel Like?

Oh, I know you don't want to go there. But just like the powerful positive reinforcement you gained on your perfect posture *visual* journey, the negative reinforcement of *feeling* poor posture might be equally as motivating. These are the exact symptoms my physical therapy patients, from weekend warriors to professional football players in the NFL, have described to me over the past 35 years. Let's give it a try.

Let's jump back into the powerful first-person role to see poor standing and sitting posture through our own eyes. To reinforce what we now know about perfect posture, let's briefly step across the dreaded line to see how painful and limiting poor posture can be. If, right now, you were living with chronic poor posture, the following sections describe what you might be feeling.

Neck and upper back symptoms

>> The back base of your skull where your neck meets your upper back is tight and achy.

>> Your neck feels super-stiff and painful when you turn your head to look over your shoulder while backing your car out of the driveway.

>> A throbbing and burning sensation screams from the base of your neck to your elbow when you fall asleep in a bad position.

>> After you've been looking down at your computer or phone for a mere ten minutes, your lower neck seems to cramp.

>> Your upper trapezius muscle, where your neck meets your upper back, is tight as a rock 24/7.

Shoulder symptoms

If you have poor posture, you may feel it in your shoulders in the following ways:

» You can't get comfortable while you sleep lying on either side because of shoulder pain.

» Reaching for anything in front or to the side, like a container of milk in the refrigerator or a bag in the back seat of your car, produces a sharp, stabbing pain deep in the front of your shoulder.

» Your chest feels overly tight, while the back of your shoulder feels overly weak.

» Reaching for anything overhead, regardless of its weight, is painful and disheartening.

Lower back symptoms

Poor posture may also manifest in your lower back with the following symptoms:

» Lower back pain can be crippling if you bend too much or lift something too heavy.

» The constant lower back tightness, which extends across the top of your butt cheeks, never seems to go away.

» Your hamstrings are constantly tight, and you just know it has to do with your chronic back problems.

» After sitting for as little as ten minutes, you have to stand and walk around.

» The numbness in the side of your hip and down your leg feels like a bad toothache.

» At times, your foot feels numb and weak.

» The risk of making your lower back worse is too great to even consider going to the gym or exercising at home.

Improving Your Posture

PT NOTE

When it comes to improving your posture, don't try to fix every issue at the same time. Focus on the painful regions. Poor posture puts unnecessary stress on parts of your body that weren't designed to bear the new stress.

Here are some examples:

>> A forward head makes the muscles of your upper back work overtime to keep your head up.

>> A forward head forces the upper cervical (neck) spine to hyperextend at the back base of the skull, putting high stress on ligaments, muscles and nerves in that area. This is an area closely associated with migraine headaches.

>> Forward, rounded shoulders limits shoulder girdle range of motion forcing your shoulder joints to work harder.

>> Forward, rounded shoulders allow the chest pec muscles to become overly tight which reinforces a tight and painful thoracic spine.

>> Exaggerated lumbar spine curve results in weak abdominal muscles and high compression on the lower back discs and bones.

TIP

Here are a few tips to help you improve your posture:

>> **Start at the top.** Tuck in your chin to park it over your ribs. The average head weighs 11 pounds. If your 11-pound melon is hanging in front of your ribs all day, your entire spine is working hard to compensate. Reel it back, Mr. Potato Head.

>> **Unlock tight muscles.** Use your rollers and roller balls to unlock your tight muscles. Typical poor posture culprits include the pectoralis minor of the chest, hip flexors, and latissimus dorsi over your kidneys.

>> **Shorten weak muscles.** Balance your body by waking up weak posture-important muscles. Typical reloaders on a poor-posture body include the rhomboid muscles between your shoulder blades, gluteal butt muscles, and lower abdominal muscles.

>> **Use the new you.** When you gain any ground with improved posture, get up and move! You want to re-educate your body to move and maintain this new posture-enhanced you. Use the new posture, new flexibility, and new strength to help your body create a new default baseline. "Hey body, there's a new enhanced sheriff in town, so ya better get used to it!"

>> **Stretch your limits.** With new posture come new muscle and joint motions. Start stretching more. Expand your movements with even the little things you do to help you maintain your new posture. For example, readjust your car mirrors for a perfect sitting posture; reach higher when washing your armpits in the shower; and step up to every other step when you walk up the stairs to bed at night.

» **Strengthen your core.** Core strength is key for so many reasons beyond posture. Find ways to include core exercises while maintaining great posture. Balance exercises help your core muscles and should be a part of your daily To Do list. It can be as simple as standing on one foot while waiting at the elevator, hopping barefoot in the grass from foot to foot, or doing a single-leg stand on a pillow with your eyes closed during commercials while watching your favorite nightly comedy show.

» **Be kind to your spine.** A strong spine is a happy spine, and every spine needs some TLC. Show those 24 vertebral bones between your sacrum and your skull some love. Slouching on a soft couch, a soft abdomen, and constantly bending over with straight legs is killing your back! If you don't think those three things are a big deal, just ask someone you know who has chronic lower back pain. When you do, look closely at their eyes. They will probably start getting teary-eyed because they would give anything to be where you are now: living with a happy spine. Now is the time to spend some time taking care of your spine while you still can.

Chapter **12**

How Muscles and Joints (Supposedly) Work in Harmony

The human body in motion is the ultimate symphony. The simple act of walking requires repetitive contractions of over 600 muscles, nerve impulses traveling at 260 miles per hour, all four chambers of the heart pumping six quarts of blood per minute, and the brain subconsciously coordinating important To Do's like posture, sweating, balance, eye motion and, oh yeah, breathing.

In this chapter, I share perspective on why view your body as truly the ultimate machine. You discover how all eleven systems in your body work together to keep you safe, healthy, and active mostly on autopilot, requiring only minor input from you. Then, to bring your body-function journey back to the rollers, you look inside your muscles and joints, seeing how the two work together in harmony. And to keep this topic real, we'll marvel how your muscles and joints seamlessly compensate when faced with injury or dysfunction. Having a better understanding of how muscles and joints are expected to function in a healthy manner will make your rolling goals much clearer and easier to achieve.

Your Body — The Ultimate Machine

When we watch a highly skilled athlete like the NFL's Patrick Mahomes or the NBA's LeBron James play, their movements look effortless and graceful, as shown in Figure 12-1. Yet when we understand what takes place under their skin to generate those complicated movements, it showcases how impressive the human body truly is.

Your body is a complex machine made up of 11 main systems.

>> **Skeletal system:** Provides the body's structural framework

>> **Muscular system:** Helps the body move

>> **Nervous system:** Collects information from receptors and the brain to coordinate cell function throughout the body

>> **Cardiovascular (circulatory) system:** Circulates blood to body organs and cells

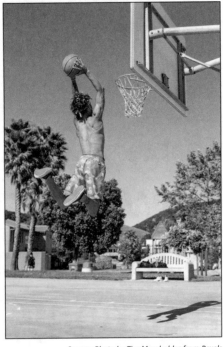

Source: Photo by Tim Mossholder from Pexels

FIGURE 12-1:
Athletic movements with effortless grace and precision.

>> **Respiratory system:** Brings oxygen into the lungs while removing carbon dioxide

>> **Digestive system:** Absorbs needed nutrients from ingested food then eliminates waste products from the gastrointestinal tract

>> **Lymphatic system:** Protects the body from harmful pathogens while draining extremities of waste products

>> **Urinary system:** Removes waste products from the blood through the kidneys and into the bladder

>> **Endocrine system:** Secretes chemical signals, allowing other body systems to respond to changes in the environment as well as between systems

>> **Reproductive system:** System responsible for childbirth

>> **Integumentary system:** The skin, hair, nails, and assorted glands help protect the body against infection, abrasion, and excessive heat

The brain communicates with the body with a reported 100,000 chemical reactions *every* second! The complexity and efficiency of the human body, as shown in Figure 12-2, is fascinating. And the human body's ability to instantly coordinate the function of all 11 of its systems at extraordinary speeds makes the human body, in my opinion, the eighth wonder of the world.

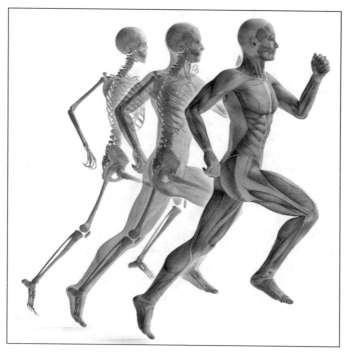

FIGURE 12-2: The human body is the ultimate machine.

adike/Shutterstock

PT NOTE

One of the most fascinating elements of the body's ability to function on such a grand scale is the fact that it can do so much at a subconscious level. The brain is able to coordinate an unfathomable number of body functions behind the scenes, so to speak, without bothering us with the details. The brain and the body have learned exactly what's needed to get the job done, and they simply do it.

Here's a simple example of how the brain and body work together. Let's say you decide to ride your bike to the park. Your brain quickly kicks into gear. With very little conscious thought on your part, your brain and body seamlessly coordinate the necessary functions with your body systems required to safely ride your bike:

>> Coordinate the necessary muscle contractions and balance to get on your bike.

>> Initiate bilateral hand-grip strength and leg-muscle strength on the pedals.

>> Coordinate core stability and inner-ear vestibular feedback to balance on the bike seat.

>> Coordinate eye motion and defensive eye-tracking skills to steer clear of danger.

>> Increase your heart rate and blood pumping volume per contraction.

>> Increase your skin's sweat rate to dissipate heat during the upcoming exercise.

>> Increase your breathing rate for an elevated demand for oxygen.

This is just a fraction of what your brain and body will do, even before you leave your driveway on your bike.

REMEMBER

The bottom line is your body and brain are fascinating. You need to appreciate your body and your brain to ensure that you properly care for them. Taking proper care of this intricate machine is so important. This means proper fueling, necessary maintenance, promptly making repairs when it is damaged, using it as it was designed to be used, and maximizing its recovery after it's been stressed.

PT NOTE

I think it's sad that most people seem to know and understand the inner workings of their smartphones better than they do their own body. It's my professional quest to change that attitude with everyone I meet. Will you join me by being the next person to make the change? Do you want to gain a simple yet rewarding understanding of how your muscles and joints work together? I surely hope your answer is "yes."

Understanding How Healthy Muscles and Joints Work Together

Healthy muscles and healthy joints are made for each other. They communicate with each other in perfect harmony. Joint receptors throughout your joint capsules and surrounding structures like bone, ligaments, and fascia are constantly feeding data to your brain. Your skeletal muscles have a tendon on each end attaching them to a bone. The muscle communicates with your brain with the help of your Golgi tendon organs (Figure 12-3) located in your muscle tendons and your muscle spindles (Figure 12-4) scattered throughout your skeletal muscles. These two types of receptors provide your brain with tons of feedback related to each of those muscles and their tendons.

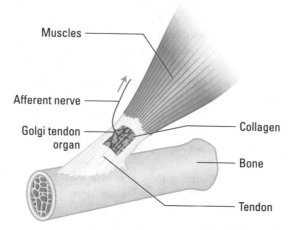

FIGURE 12-3:
Golgi tendon organs located in the anchoring tendons for each muscle.

Muscles

Afferent nerve

Golgi tendon organ

Collagen

Bone

Tendon

©John Wiley & Sons, Inc.

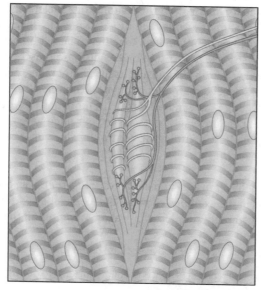

FIGURE 12-4:
Muscle spindles are stretch receptors in skeletal muscle.

Dorling Kindersley/Getty Images

Your brain functions like a military command center, sharing all this information with relevant joints and muscles as well as other vital organs, like the eyes for vision and the inner ear for balance.

REMEMBER

Why is information important for you as a roller? Understanding how your muscle (tendon-muscle-tendon) works with your brain will help you work with your muscle when it is both healthy and dysfunctional. For example, reflect back to a time when one of your muscles was injured or was dysfunctional because of a painful trigger point or cramp. You quickly noticed the muscle seemed to have a mind of its own and regardless what you and your brain told it to do, the muscle "went rogue" and remained tight and semi-contracted. That's an example of the muscle receptors, Golgi tendon organs, and muscle spindles sending mixed messages to the brain because of the injury or trigger point in the muscles. By using a roller or roller ball to relax a tight or semi-contracted muscle, the stress on the tendon-muscle-tendon structure is reduced and the receptors can return to sending clear messages to the brain. When a muscle is relaxed following a roller treatment, the muscle fibers, its tendons, and the busy surrounding fascia return to their looser status and have improved function.

With every step, your brain instantly knows where its body weight is dissipated, which muscles to contract, which muscles are stretching, and every joint angle. It also knows the location of every instantaneous sensation like pressure, numbness, fascia stretch, and good old-fashioned pain.

PT NOTE

The structure of the skeletal, or striated, muscle is important for you to know. (Refer to Chapter 10 for an image of the anatomy of a skeletal muscle.) Put simply, each muscle is made up of a collection of small muscle fibers. Those individual muscle fibers are wrapped, or bundled, together in large numbers, surrounded by fascia like a spaghetti-filled burrito. Bundles of these muscle fibers are grouped together with fascia to form the muscle itself. The number, position, angle, and length of the fibers depend on the function of the muscle. Stronger, thicker muscles found in your thigh have more fibers with more powerful functions, such as jumping and running. Conversely, muscles in your hand have smaller numbers of fibers with more intricate neurological control for finer, more accurate functions like writing and painting.

Let's take a look at how muscles and joints work together in a perfect world within a perfect body. As in the example, consider the legs as they perform the simple act of walking. The seemingly simple act of walking requires all the following steps:

1. One hundred percent of the bodyweight is shifted to the left leg.

2. The right hip flexor contracts concentrically (shortens) to pull the right leg forward.

3. The right hamstring slowly contracts eccentrically (lengthens) to slow the forward swinging motion of the right leg.

4. As the right heel hits the ground, the right quad muscle contracts eccentrically to absorb the force of the right leg impacting the ground.

5. As the center of gravity shifts from the left leg towards the right leg, the body weight is quickly shifted to the right leg.

6. The right anterior tibialis muscle located in the front of the shin contracts eccentrically to lower the right foot to a flat position on the ground.

7. The dozens of little muscles located in the right foot and arch quickly kick into gear to stabilize the entire right lower extremity, which is being slammed down into the arch, resulting in a force on the sole of the foot of approximately 2000 pounds per square inch.

8. The quad muscles contract concentrically to straighten out the knee.

9. The stability of the right leg is now a high priority because the left leg is now off the ground and swinging forward.

10. All three glute muscles, all six groin muscles, the six hip rotators, the three hamstring muscles, all the fascia throughout the entire right lower extremity, and the two calf muscles work together to generate the necessary type of muscle contraction (concentric, eccentric, and isometric) to stabilize the moving leg under the moving body.

11. With the left leg now contacting the ground, the right three glute muscles kick into gear and generate a strong, concentric contraction to hold the right thigh backwards in relation to the pelvis.

12. With the angle of the ankle now changing, the two calf muscles contract concentrically to raise the right heel, shifting the entire weight of the right leg to the front of the right foot.

13. With the entire right arch and right toe flexor muscles placed in an extremely flexed position, the fascia from the tips of the right toes all the way up to the right hamstring is stretched and loaded.

14. To propel the body weight back to the left leg, a highly coordinated and timely concentric contraction of the right glutes, hamstrings, and calf muscles takes place.

15. With the entire bodyweight now shifted to the left leg, the shin anterior tibialis muscle, right hamstring, and right hip flexor all contract concentrically, allowing the right foot to clear the ground as it swings forward.

PT NOTE

Now imagine how fast these key steps of motion need to take place when an athlete is running fast, changing directions involving her entire body on uneven ground, and tracking a speeding ball in the air, while avoiding other fast-moving athletes.

Knowing When Your Body Needs a Wheel Alignment

In the previous section, I talked about how your muscles and joints all synchronize when everything is perfect and every system is working flawlessly. Let's look at what happens when your muscles and joints are less than perfect. For instance,

>> How does an overly tight hamstring muscle and fascia change the way your knee extends?

>> How does an arthritic knee with bone spurs and limited knee bend impact your lower back when you run?

>> How does your brain alter the firing pattern of your rotator cuff muscles when your shoulder joint is limited in motion because of a chronic labral tear?

REMEMBER

These examples are much less pretty compared to the perfect body example from the previous section. But the reality for probably 95 percent of us is located in this section of the book. What I mean by that is most of us have some type of limitation involving our muscles or joints. Because of our past medical history, occupation, age, activity level, sport, posture, flexibility, core strength, moving patterns, extremity strength, sitting habits, balance, and attitude, we're forced to alter the way we move.

Compensating to keep moving

So, what happens when your body has to alter its movement patterns? Your body and brain just find a way to get the job done, period. That's right, your body and brain just go to option B — or C or Z, if needed — to meet your moving objective. Simply stated, your body compensates. The skills your body and brain demonstrate during situations when your body is limited in motion and in pain may be more impressive than what you see with the perfectly functioning body. Your body certainly is a perfect compensating machine. The following table provides some common examples of orthopedic compensations.

Limitation	Compensation
Reduced shoulder joint elevation	Increased shoulder girdle elevation
Reduced balance	Wider feet placement when walking
Limited neck extension	Increased upper neck hyperextension
Rounded, tight shoulders	Lumbar hyperextension (sway back)

Limitation	Compensation
Lumbar degenerative discs	Forward shoulders and head
Arthritic hip	Increased hip external rotation
Arthritic knee	Flexion contracture of hamstrings
Knee-bone spurs	Increased muscle tone of calf muscles
Collapsed arches	Hyperflexion of big toe

PT NOTE

When limited in motion or in pain, your body and brain simply divert to your backup owner's manual to find a way to compensate. It's fascinating how effective your body becomes in order to meet your objective, yet most of this process is still invisible. Your brain "keeps its eyes on the prize," which is your desired movement or activity, and it simply works around your limitations and deficiencies.

Looking at long-term consequences of altered movement

The difficult question is what will the long-term results of these changes be? Obviously, these compensations and mechanical changes mean that your body will pay a price. The longer the body compensations take place, the higher the cost.

Scenario 1: Temporary pain

Consider this first scenario: Suppose you're late getting your son RollerBaby to school one morning. You realize you have a rock in your shoe, but you don't have time to stop, so you walk the 400 yards to school with the rock still in your shoe. Your body and brain recognize the negative stimulus (pain) and simply alter the way you move (compensation). Because the pain is not perceived as significantly dangerous, your body simply compensates due to the pain associated with that rock.

Leaving the school with RollerBaby safely in his classroom, you simply pluck the rock from your shoe. As easily as you removed the rock from your shoe, your walking pattern returns to normal. The change was temporary. No damage was done.

Scenario 2: Long-term pain

Now take the very same example as Scenario 1, but instead of the source of your foot pain coming from the small rock, it's coming from a painful, bony bunion and arthritis at the ball of your foot. Like Scenario 1, you'll probably still limp as you bring your son to school. But obviously the source of your pain is not temporary, and it cannot be removed quickly. Therefore, the way your body compensates will remain altered for your joints and muscles both above and below your limited and painful joint.

Scenario 3: Scar tissue and compensation

Another way to look at this can be demonstrated with a 15-foot piece of steel-link chain. If you wrap the link chain around a large tree, each one of those chain links bend between each other. Think of the connections between each link as a joint. They could represent your hip joint, knee joint, or the joints between the vertebral bones of your spine. Next, to replicate the restrictive nature of scar tissue or tight fascia, you tightly wrap duct tape around five of those chain links. Afterwards, you can still wrap the chain around the tree. But, when you look at the five links, or joints, with the duct tape around them, you notice that the joints are tight and restricted and obviously have less motion between them.

Joint compensation and posture

Now look at the joints just before and just after the duct tape. What do you notice most about those joints (connection between 2 chain links)? Can you see how they are forced to demonstrate much more motion? It's easy to visualize the extra stress and motion placed on the joints on both sides of the tight and restricted (taped) joints. What you're seeing is these joints having to compensate with extra motion and stress.

REMEMBER

This is how the body works: It goes into "just get 'er done" mode. But when the body does this, extra stress and load are placed on parts of the body that are not designed for the increased demands.

PT NOTE

With altered body mechanics, due to anything from tight muscles to weak muscles to an injury, some body parts are overloaded while others are underloaded. Overloaded body parts can lead to overuse injuries, stress fracture, strains, tendonitis, inflammation, and pain.

OUCH

Meanwhile, other body parts may be underloaded and prone to not work so hard. Such a change can be equally problematic. For example, poor head and shoulder posture, as shown in Figure 12-5, forces muscles in the chest and back of the neck to be shortened and overly tight. Conversely, the now-rounded shoulders result in the spreading apart of the shoulder blades. The result: weak and underloaded stabilizing muscles between the shoulder blades and overloaded thoracic spine ligaments being "hung on" when sitting in a slumped posture.

OUCH

Staying with this common poor-posture dilemma, the head is forced significantly forward in front of the ribs, forcing the muscles on the front of the neck to be underloaded and weak. Conversely, the muscles on the back of the neck are forced to work overtime just to keep the eleven-pound head up. (I've seen plenty of NFL heads that weighed much more than eleven pounds!) It's not a coincidence when these individuals with forward head posture complain about having very tight muscles at the base of their necks. In fact, it's common to hear them use the expression, "I carry my stress in my neck."

Because the human body is so accurately designed, random changes are not always good. For example, an arthritic knee results in a reduced range of motion. So, the brain says: "Hey, listen up, right leg. We have a painful knee on board with a lot of wear and tear. It doesn't feel well today so, hey, right hip, I need you to do some extra pulling and right ankle, tighten up 'cuz I need 30 percent more plantar flexion push from you, stat! We need to work together to help get this poor knee through the day."

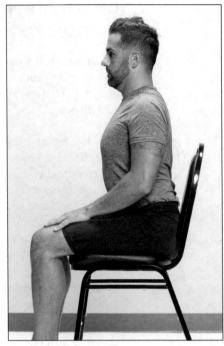

Photography by Haim Ariav & Klara Cu

FIGURE 12-5:
Poor posture changes the role of muscles, joints, and fascia.

Well, that may sound like a great plan, and it will get you through the day. But after weeks and months on this compensation plan, the right quad muscle doesn't have much of a workload, so it decides to go on vacation. As a result, the right quad becomes atrophied and weak while the right hamstring becomes overworked and super-tight.

Meanwhile, the overworked right hip flexor becomes painful, which forces the glutes to join the quads on the chillin' vacation. The sudden lower-extremity change overloads the hip rotators and the calf muscles, which now have to work overtime. With the hip flexors, hip rotators, and calf muscles overworked and desperately needing some time off, the entire lower back locks up in angry protest to support its friends in the southern neighborhood. Needless to say, in a compensation cycle like this, things (muscles, joints, fascia, tendons, ligaments, and so on) can get ugly and painful very quickly.

Identifying pain and limitations in order to fix them

Compensations are okay for a short period of time. But it should be a high priority for you to keep your muscles, fascia, and joints moving as they were designed to move, with bilateral symmetry. If you can do this, you will keep moving pain-free and with ease.

PT NOTE

I love my job and my profession as a physical therapist and certified athletic trainer because I have the privilege of being entrusted by others to care for their most treasured possession: their *health*. I have learned so much about the human body and its capabilities by listening to my patients, and to my own body. Understanding their true limitations and the source of their pain is extremely important for me and for the health of my patients. I'm very good at asking my patients specific questions to get honest, clear answers regarding their key limitations and the core source of their pain. Here are some examples:

>> **What is your number one limitation?** Understanding and addressing what *they*, not me or their doctor or spouse, perceived as their number one problem is paramount.

>> **What is the source (or sources) of your pain?** Eliminating their pain, regardless of how intense it may be, cannot happen if the source is not properly identified.

It all comes down to this simple question: How can you positively influence your body's limitations without surgery or medicine to help you move better?

PT NOTE

It's been my experience as a physical therapist, certified athletic trainer, and certified Spartan SGX coach and athlete, that many of the factors that force people to move abnormally can be positively changed by unlocking overly tight muscles and improving joint range of motion. Please believe me, your solution for pain-free motion can be that simple.

This is where the rollers are worth their weight in gold. With the detailed treatment plans in this book, your rollers will keep your muscles, fascia, and joints tuned up and ready to happily do their job. Rollers to the rescue!

I hope that news gets you excited. With the help of this book and a moderate amount of time on your part, positive changes are coming for your body that will involve less pain throughout a wider range of motion.

Now that is something worth celebrating!

impact on our bodies and how
we move

» Applying tips to work with our
fascia instead of working against
our fascia

» Mobilizing dysfunctional fascia as
an important part of roller therapy

Chapter **13**

Fascia: Taming the Beast

ascia is Latin for bandage or band, and it is categorized as a connective tissue. Made of elastin fibers, which allow it to stretch, and collagen, which provides its strength, fascia is similar to a spider's web. It is composed of tiny tubules containing fluid, which allows for three-dimensional mobility, and is covered with a gel-like material.

I'm a big fan of fascia — also referred to as myofascial connective tissue because of its strong involvement with muscle tissue. And when fascia is managed properly, or "tamed" if you will, I consider it to be the most underappreciated tissue in the human body.

How Tight Fascia Makes Even Simple Movements Hard

Take a moment to look at Figure 13-1. This complex, yet beautiful, connective tissue is scattered throughout your entire body like wild ivy vine engulfing a small tree in a field. If you "tame" your fascia with effective roller treatments and stretching, the fascial vine functions like little rubber bands gently hugging the tree as it effortlessly sways in the breeze. In contrast, if you don't tame your fascial vine, the fascial fibers become tight and restrictive resulting in the fascial vine functioning like a web of leather straps tightly strangling the helpless tree.

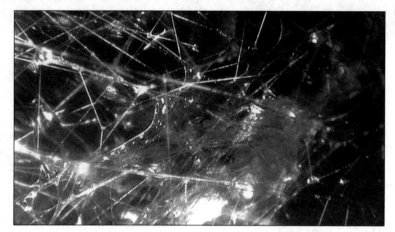

FIGURE 13-1:
The beauty, complexity, and strength of the human body's fascial web.

J.C. Guimberteau M.D/ENDOVIVO Video Productions

REMEMBER

With fascia's massive size and all-encompassing landscape around almost every-structure in your body from the tips of your toes to the top of your head, every movement involves your fascia. Even the simple act of breathing is impacted by your body's fascia. So, keeping your fascia mobile and flexible is a high priority if you want to move with minimal restrictions.

There are many reasons why fascia becomes restricted and limits motion in your body. Fascia can be difficult to treat because it may be restricted by a tight trigger point or scar tissue in one area of your body, resulting in symptoms in a different part of your body.

The following example is something we can all relate to.

PT NOTE

Let's assume your shirt represents the fascia surrounding your ribs and abdomen. Tuck your shirt into your pants extra deep and tight. Now stand with your hands at your sides. Any problems? Probably not. Now walk around the room. You're probably still fine. The restricted lower shirt seems fine, with no impact on your standing or walking. Now I want you to simply reach one hand for the sky. How's the tight lower shirt moving now?

The simple act of flexing one joint is impacted by restricted fascia (your lower shirt) over two feet away! Now imagine if you sewed your pants and shirt together, much like tight scar tissue or a trigger point would do, and you played tennis or swam with such a limitation. It would be easy to see how your shoulder, spine, ribs, abdominals, and pelvis would be forced to move differently, or compensate, because of the bound-down fascial web in your mid-section.

OUCH

Here are some reasons for fascial restrictions:

>> **Surgery:** The act of cutting, removing, or suturing skin and underlying tissue

>> **Overuse:** Too much activity

>> **Trauma:** Excessive external force

>> **Infection:** Insult to tissue

>> **Repetitive motion:** Very limited motion with little deviation to stretch tissue

>> **Dysfunctional breathing:** Abnormal diaphragm, abdomen, and rib function

>> **Poor posture:** Prolonged sitting at a computer, carrying a heavy backpack, slumping while standing at a standup desk

>> **Inflammation:** Result of dysfunction of tissue

>> **Lack of activity or motion:** Sedentary or minimal total-body motion

>> **Tight muscles:** Restricted muscles, which equals restricted surrounding fascia

>> **Emotional stress:** A factor that impacts the dynamics of fascia

>> **Leg length discrepancy:** Incompatibility that results in bilateral dissymmetry

>> **High volume of unilateral activities:** One-sided functions (like throwing, painting, and kicking) that strengthen and stretch one side of the body much differently than the other side

>> **Dysfunctional body mechanics:** Lack of bilateral symmetry because of poor muscle contraction patterns

>> **Chronically tight fascia:** Tight, inflexible fascia that tends to cinch down and restrict motion of everything in its neighborhood

>> **Restrictive adhesions:** Tight scar tissue that can reduce the normal mobility of surrounding fascia and muscle

That's a long list. The reason why there are so many factors impacting the function of fascia is two-fold.

>> **Size:** Fascial tissue is intertwined with so many different types of tissue. Reflecting back to the wild ivy vine story at the beginning of the section, that vine is now impacted by any changes to the tree trunk, bark, large branches, small branches, and leaves. Now if your body is wrapped in inelastic, limiting fascia, as your muscles expand and grow, as they normally do with healthy exercise, the restrictions from the tightened fascia become tighter! See Figure 13-2.

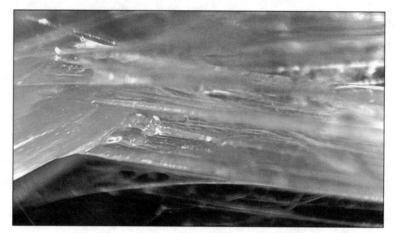

FIGURE 13-2:
Fascia is tightly wrapped around almost all of your muscles, joints, and bones.

J.C. Guimberteau M.D/ENDOVIVO Video Productions

>> **Mobility:** Fascial tissue's ability to slide and move in a three-dimensional manner allows it to apply stress to areas of the body far away from any localized injury or adhesion.

PT NOTE

What's restricting the fascia or muscle? It can involve many factors, as you read in the previous sections. Many believe the restriction comes from a simple adhesion. An adhesion is defined as "the action or process of adhering to a surface."

In your body, you have many layers of "stuff" that slide over each other like your clothes move over your body as you move. Your jacket is separate from your shirt, pants, and underwear. Now introduce a small adhesion. Let's have fun with this example.

Let's assume you have a tube of SuperDuper Glue in your pants pocket, and it starts to leak. It glues your pants to your favorite pair of superhero underwear. It now slightly changes how your pants and underwear all work together. "It's not a big deal," you say, "I'll clean it up when I get home."

Suddenly, the glue leak gets worse and now your jacket, shirt, pants, and super-hero undies are glued together solid as a rock! It's still in the same area as before, but now the adhesion encompasses more layers. Now you walk differently. Your hip and spine motion are altered. Your emotions are different, too. You worry about how you'll sit at your desk, drive your car, get undressed, and if anyone will notice how you move. Now this "It's not a big deal" has become a big problem!

Can you now see how even small, localized adhesions can impact the function of both your body and your mind?

Tight Fascia's Impact on Other Types of Tissue

Now you know the many reasons why fascia can become restricted. When this fascial web loses any of its three-dimensional mobility, any of the different types of tissue, including muscles, joints, blood vessels, nerves, lymphatic vessels, or organs, are also prone to lose mobility as well.

REMEMBER

If your fascia is properly aligned and mobile like a well-fitted pair of stretchy leg tights, it allows the muscles and joints to be mobile and powerful. But if your fascial web loses its normal mobility from, say, a tight adhesion that formed from the trauma of a recent painful fall, that same fascia is now restrictive like a pair of wet, tight jeans. This new tight fascia will now make your muscles and joints feel stiff and weak.

OUCH

Restricted fascia symptoms include the following:

>> Tight and bound-down skin

>> Headache

>> Breathing difficulties

>> Numbness or tingling in arms or legs

>> Recurring soft tissue injuries

>> General body pain

>> Hot or burning pain in your torso or extremities

>> Generalized lower back ache

>> Chronic joint or muscle stiffness

>> Clumsiness and uncoordinated body movements

>> Limited joint range of motion

>> Muscle knots

>> Muscle cramps

>> Dull, hot, aching muscle pain

>> Aching leg or arm

>> Poor posture

>> Poor flexibility of extremity

Tips for Healthy Fascia

"Hey dude, how's your fascia feeling?" may not be a common greeting between you and your friends. But it should be. Keeping your fascia healthy will be a much higher priority for you after reading this book.

>> **Pinching yourself.** Find areas on your body where the skin seems to be anchored down too tightly. Pinch the skin and try to pull it away from the underlying muscle at different angles. Fascia is known to bind skin down to the underlying tissue such as fat, muscle, or bone. After pinching and pulling the skin away in different directions, compare the treated skin's mobility to the same location on the other side of your body.

>> **Keep on rolling.** Consistently use a roller above, below, and on areas of tightness.

>> **Drink.** Stay well hydrated, especially with water.

>> **Stretch.** Include low-intensity, long-duration stretches in your flexibility routine.

>> **Police patrol.** Always assess your body for areas that seem bound down and overly taut.

>> **Stretch above and below.** When rolling and stretching, make a habit of changing joint positions both above and below the roller or stretch. For example, when stretching your hamstrings, change the position of your ankle joint. As another example, when rolling your chest muscles, change your head and elbow positions to see how they alter the treatment of your chest.

>> **Massage.** A more superficial massage, which mobilizes the skin and the fascia just under the skin, should be part of your fascia maintenance plan. This is very different from a deeper, aggressive "sports massage," which focuses on the deeper power muscles.

Dysfunctional fascia happens frequently in our ever-changing bodies with our ever-changing body positions in our ever-changing busy schedules. It's typically when those fascial restrictions become excessive or prolonged that other systems become involved and the body is forced to divert to significant compensations.

A small, temporary adhesion resulting in a minor tightness of a muscle or a tight knee capsule is no reason to call 911. But if that adhesion becomes tighter and painful, resulting in a consistent limp, and the overloaded muscles develop large, painful trigger points, then the story is very different.

PT NOTE

This is where a consistent maintenance plan involving your rollers is so valuable. It helps you police your body for early signs of mild issues before they become major problems. The assessment plans and treatment protocols in this book will help you find and extinguish small, smoking brush fires before they become a major forest fire.

Chapter **14**

Managing Scar Tissue

S car tissue has a bad reputation in the minds of most people. But when you talk to athletic trainers, physical therapists, massage therapists, surgeons, and other manual therapists who work with soft tissue injuries, you quickly learn the value of *healthy* scar tissue. I hope you noticed that I referenced "healthy scar tissue"; unhealthy or dysfunctional scar tissue, on the other hand, can be a living nightmare for its host.

In this chapter I give you an honest and clear look at scar tissue and how to manage it. You can never completely avoid scar tissue because it's part of the normal healing process throughout your body. The role of scar tissue is to close the gap between injured tissue. Therefore, the complete absence of scar tissue would be disastrous.

What Is Scar Tissue?

When normal tissue is injured, the human body immediately kicks into healing mode. The damage to the tissue can come in many forms, such as trauma, overuse, surgery, or disease. Regardless of the source of the insult, the body recognizes that tissue damage has occurred and quickly starts the repair process.

As the wound bleeding starts to slow and the cellular damage is stabilized, the body begins the mechanical steps necessary to close the gaps within or between the injured tissue. It starts with the process of pulling the sides of the injury site back together.

A simple example is a laceration on the back of your hand. Once the bleeding stops, a thin scab forms on top of the wound and the depth of the wound begins to reduce as the floor of the laceration is raised. Next, the two sides of the cut are pulled closer to each other.

The scab, or filler, is a form of scar tissue. Although it may not look like it to begin with, scar tissue is composed of the same protein (collagen) as the body tissue it's replacing on either side of the scar.

Of course, the scar tissue's characteristics are usually quite different. The collagen fibers in the new scar tissue tend to have a different fiber alignment and pattern than the same type of collagen found in the surrounding tissue. Because of this alteration of the new collagen fibers, the scar tissue functions differently than the tissue it's replacing. In other words, scar tissue does a great job of filling in the injury holes, but that same tissue moves differently than the surrounding tissue.

PT NOTE

Case in point: When I was a kid and my favorite jeans got a hole in the knee, my loving and resourceful mother would iron a jean patch over the hole. The patch did a stellar job of covering the hole and protecting the damaged denim cloth around the hole. My mother's plan was to repair the hole and prevent the denim around it from continuing to fray and tear. Mission accomplished, Mom!

But when I returned to my legendary life of playground mayhem, the knee patch clearly didn't have the same stretch, mobility, or "feel" as the denim around my other knee. That's similar to scar tissue in the body. Scar tissue usually does its job, but the end result is typically a tighter and more restrictive tissue.

REMEMBER

When I reference a scar, it doesn't have to mean a cut or scrape involving the skin. A scar and the resulting scar tissue can be located in the skin, just under the skin, deep inside a muscle, in a joint capsule, or anywhere in between. Any body tissue, from your toes to your head, is susceptible to an injury. Therefore, healing scar tissue can be found anywhere in your body.

Four Phases of Scar Healing

Understanding how your body heals will help you better influence your healing with rollers, roller balls, handheld massagers and vibrating rollers. This is where the "art" of rolling comes into play. Another way to look at this is to find ways to enhance the body's ability to progress through these four phases of scar healing quickly without regressing or going backwards.

1. **Stopping the "madness."** The first phase stops the bleeding using blood platelets and thrombin to form stable clots in the area of damage.

2. **Cleanup time.** The inflammation phase removes debris and bacteria to prepare the lesion for the arrival of the new tissue.

3. **Filling in the holes.** The proliferation phase adds new, healthy collagen, narrowing the opening and covering the wound.

4. **Maturing the scar.** The remodeling phase occurs when the collagen fibers stretch and strengthen, while trying to match the abilities of the tissue surrounding the wound.

As you can see in Figure 14-1, with a simple lesion involving injured skin tissue, the healing process both protects and closes the damaged tissue. Scar tissue is the glue used by the body to patch the injured tissue together.

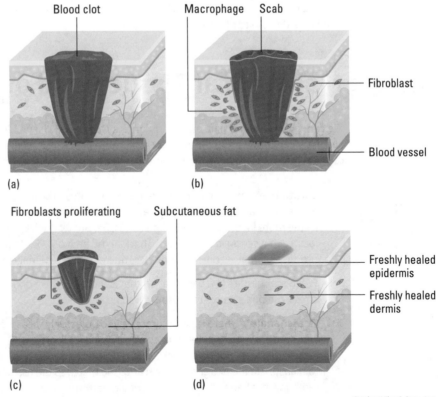

FIGURE 14-1: The four steps to healing a wound.

© John Wiley & Sons, Inc.

THE GOOD SIDE OF A SCAR

When we get hurt, scar tissue has a dirty job to do. Even after the healing, scar tissue is looked down upon if there's any question that it's the source of the pain. It's safe to say that scar tissue is in a less-than-admirable position.

But don't let the bad rap cloud your personal opinion of scar tissue. It serves an important role in fixing parts of our body that have been damaged. It's available 24/7 to adapt to almost any type of tissue protein (collagen).

"We *want* scar tissue on that wound. We *need* scar tissue on that wound!

Now imagine a more complicated setting for scar tissue to work its magic. Let's use the bottom of your heel as an example, with a painful injury known as plantar fasciitis. Unlike the simple example shown in Figure 14-1, healing swollen and painful scar tissue located in the arch of your foot is a much harder task.

To better understand the value of a healthy scar, let's take a closer look at the good and bad sides of scar tissue.

Factors Making Scar Tissue Good or Bad

We can't list all scar tissue on either Santa's Good Scar Tissue List or Bad Scar Tissue list. Scar tissue has an important job. There are certain traits or characteristics of scar tissue which determine if that particular scar tissue is either friend or foe.

PT NOTE

>> **Location.** An important factor related to the status of scar tissue can be applied to real estate: location, location, location. Hopefully, by now you have a little more love in your heart for scar tissue. But when the scar tissue is located in a sensitive area, like the back of the arch on your foot in the previous plantar fasciitis example, it's much harder to manage.

When scar tissue's in a bad location that is more sensitive or under more stress, the bad side of scar tissue will shine.

>> **"Matchability."** There is no accurate way to objectively measure how much a new scar has matched the abilities of the tissue it's replacing. Those traits include elasticity, fiber alignment, and tensile strength. But if there were a way to measure it, the better the new scar tissue matched the tissue it was replacing, the better the scar tissue would perform.

>> **Pain.** This is the easy one. The less painful the scar is, the higher the loads the injury site can tolerate.

>> **Limitations.** These tie into the "matchability" factor. The better the scar functions with the surrounding tissue, the less it limits the function of that tissue. Putting a piece of tape on a balloon is a good way to seal a hole. But the more you inflate and stretch the balloon, the greater the tape limits the function of the balloon.

Symptoms of Scar Tissue Pain

Take a look at the symptoms related to scar tissue. This list will help you pinpoint the location of the scar tissue and gauge its improvement during the recovery.

>> **Burning:** Feels hot

>> **Point tenderness:** Very localized pain or symptoms

>> **"Catching":** When tissue seems to grab or "catch" on other tissue with motion

>> **Generalized pressure:** Feels full, distended

>> **Aching:** Toothache-like

>> **Tingling and numbness:** Pins + needles, feels like the area has fallen asleep

>> **Shooting nerve pain:** Intense pain starting in one area and shooting to another location like an electrical bolt

>> **Restricted and localized tightness:** Bounded or cinched down tissue in an isolated area

I was slightly embarrassed to share this list of scar tissue symptoms because almost every one of the symptoms can apply to any other injury. Because scar tissue is a blended part of other types of tissue, compared to normal stand-alone tissue, scar tissue pain can mimic other types of tissue pain.

OUCH

When left untreated, scar tissue can disrupt body mechanics, muscle flexibility, joint range of motion, nerve conductivity, and lymphatic drainage, just to name a few. Consider a few examples of how scar tissue in certain areas can impair how otherwise healthy tissue does its job.

>> If an excessively tight scar forms in your neck muscle, entrapping a nerve, you'll experience nerve pain.

>> If an old chronic scar in a torn hamstring muscle in the back of your thigh cinches down after a four-hour car ride, you'll have the symptoms of a tight hamstring muscle.

>> After a long walk in dress shoes with the previously mentioned plantar fasciitis, you may feel fascial pain in your arch.

This is where rollers are so helpful. Early on in the healing process, rollers help keep tissues — scar tissue included — mobile and less restricted. When assessing an injury, old or new, you can use a roller to scan over tissue-busy areas of your body to help you isolate the location of the pain and restricted scar tissue. I like to think of an assessment roller as an old battlefield minesweeper. It scans the battlefield to safely find and remove deadly mines before soldiers inadvertently suffer a horrific fate when they accidentally find the mines with their feet.

PT NOTE

Another reason why scar tissue pain is not easily diagnosed is its ability to remain symptom-free for so long before becoming problematic. For reasons not completely understood, scar tissue can suddenly become painful or influence other tissues to alter their function and pain threshold. A gastrointestinal surgeon once told me about a patient of his who required emergency surgery for a complete bowel obstruction deep inside their abdomen to remove scar tissue from a previous surgery, which was completely symptom-free for 50 years!

I believe the random nature of scar tissue symptoms is based on the simple fact that soft tissue is alive and dynamic. Scar tissue is a busy area because the scar and the tissues around the scar have a blood supply, fascial support, and a nerve supply. Depending on the location and the type of tissues associated with the scar, the tissues are likely to move, stretch, contract, absorb blood, communicate with the brain, and do their assigned jobs.

Types of Scars

Not all scar tissue is created equal. Following are three common types of scar tissue. Each type possesses its own challenges for the host, especially depending on the location of the three types.

>> **Too much scar tissue.** This results in rigid and stiff collagen.

   Examples include hypertrophic scars and keloids.

>> **Sunken scar tissue.** This includes tightened collagen that blocks the completion of the collagen formation throughout the scar.

   An example is sunken scars.

>> **Stretched scar tissue.** This involves excessive stretching that elongates the scar tissue.

An example is abdominal stretch marks during pregnancy.

Now take a moment to scout your body for visible, palpable (touch), and functional (movement) restrictions potentially related to scar tissues. Do some looking, poking, tugging, sliding, stretching, twisting, squatting, and so on to find areas of restrictions. Can you see, touch, or feel something not moving like it does on the other side of your body?

Tips to Manage Scar Tissue

Remember, you don't want to eliminate scar tissue, so you simply need to properly manage it. Much like your body weight, if you manage your scar tissue properly and consistently, you'll be happy with the results.

Having managed professional football players with lots of scar tissue from multiple collisions on every play, scar tissue management became a high priority for me during my years in the NFL as an athletic trainer and physical therapist. With my largest player weighing 404 pounds, let's say large humans have a lot of real estate to host strong scar tissue. And when the scar tissue is located in an area subject to high-contact forces and repetitions, like the knee, thigh, low back, shoulder, and head, the challenges are plentiful. I want to share with you some tips for successful scar management I learned in NFL rehab rooms:

>> **Keep clean.** Thoroughly and consistently clean every wound. Dirty and infected wounds are much slower to heal, and the quality of their final scar tissue is typically inferior.

>> **Move early.** Following an injury, with the guidance of your physical therapist and doctor, start early, easy motion. It helps mobilize the lesion to promote a more flexible scar.

>> **Load light.** As with the medical guidance with early motion, applying early low-intensity loads to the injured tissue will promote a healthier scar.

>> **Keep rollin'.** Use the roller treatment plans in this book to treat scar tissue like you would trigger points. Unlocking muscles and increasing joint range of motion by quieting trigger points, scar tissue, and adhesions with rollers will accomplish the same two objectives: reducing your pain while improving your active lifestyle (see Figure 14-2).

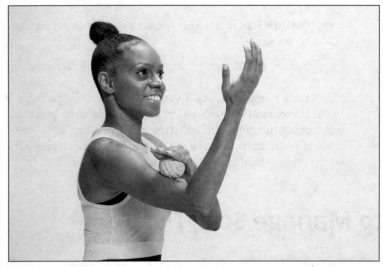

FIGURE 14-2:
Rolling to
mobilize scar
tissue.

Photography by Haim Ariav & Klara Cu

» **Mobilize the hood.** The injury may involve one localized tissue or body part. If so, get busy stretching, rolling, and exercising the muscles, tendons, joints, fascia, and ligaments in the neighborhood surrounding the injury. A soft roller on the tissue above and below the scar is a great place to start. By doing so, when your specific injury is ready to be more active, your entire body is ready to go, too.

» **Fuel healthy.** Healthy eating and drinking will supercharge your internal healing capabilities.

» **Check often.** Be diligent with consistent self-checks and medical checkups to confirm that your aggressive recovery plan is working without crossing "the line" to get re-injured.

» **Add to your routine.** When you find exercises, stretches, and rolls that promote your body's scar tissue management plan, add them into your daily maintenance routine.

4
Unlocking Tight Muscle and Fascia with Rollers

Chapter **15**

Scouting Your Body for Pain, Stiffness, and Restrictions

The first step to maximizing the benefits of rollers is to know the specific needs of your body. I want to show you simple and proven sports medicine tricks to scout your body for locations where your body is struggling with pain, stiffness, and restrictions.

In Part 4 of this book, I'll be showing you techniques to unlock your muscles and improve your range of motion. But unless you have a spare two hours every day to roll and treat your entire body, learning shortcuts to quickly find your tissues in need save you a huge amount of time.

REMEMBER

An important trait I want you to learn is the ability to listen to your body. This is a priceless skill I focus on improving in myself every day. Truly listening to my body is my number-one secret to competing and working out at a very high level with Spartan Racers half my age and still avoiding injuries.

Constructing and Interpreting Your True Past Medical History

We all have an activity history. We all have a psychological history. We all have a medical history.

When we put those three (body, mind, and medical) key elements of who we are together, we have our *true past medical history* (TPMH). I include "true" because without all three of those elements, the history of our body is not accurate — therefore, untrue.

REMEMBER

The purpose of constructing your TPMH is to start the process of building a successful, individualized maintenance plan for your body.

Why all three elements are key

I like to look at TPMH as evaluating ourselves based on our history below the neck, above the neck, and in our medical file. As shown in the following examples, your past medical history would look different if you eliminated just one of the three elements.

What if you interpreted your past medical history without including your *activity* history?

> **Result:** "I'm a nervous nelly." This is an emotional and confusing view of what your body has accomplished.

> **Why:** If you don't know your *activity history*, such as the sports you played, your body's strengths and weaknesses, or how your body responds to certain exercises, you're left looking at your past emotions and past medical setbacks. Individuals who do this have a tendency to generically reference "they" to justify why they limit themselves.

What if you interpreted your past medical history without your *psychological* history?

> **Result:** "I did that. And that. And that." This is a dreamless and shallow view of what you've accomplished physically with no emotional context as to why you did it or how you felt when you completed it.

> **Why:** If you don't know your psychological history, such as your joys and fears, why you love your active lifestyle, or the rewarding emotions you've gained when you accomplished previous big goals, then you're left simply looking at a cold, unemotional check list of accomplishments.

What if you interpreted your past medical history without your *medical* history?

Result: "I'm a dreamer." You'd be living in the past, thinking of the grand physical feats and events you did 20 years ago.

Why: If you don't know your medical history, such as previous joint injuries, past medical recommendations from physical therapists, doctors, and athletic trainers, or limiting body ailments, then you'll tend to be an injury-prone dreamer gazing at your past physical highlights.

I hope you now understand the importance of looking at your past activities, mindset, and medical care to properly evaluate your true past medical history. It only makes sense.

PT NOTE

As you know by now, I like to keep things simple and efficient. Scouting your body for pain, stiffness, and restrictions needs to be easy to do, simple to interpret, and fast with results. Those three steps are the framework of my sports medicine business.

Interpreting the information

Now that you have collected and reviewed your true past medical history, let's look at how you can best interpret that information.

REMEMBER

The reason for looking backwards at your body's history is to properly and successfully plot your active future. Without learning from your past, you increase the possibility of an injury in the future. Blindfolds are great for piñata parties, but not for planning a pain-free active lifestyle.

Complete the following steps to successfully interpret a true past medical history:

1. **List your injuries.**

We all have our bumps and bruises. The first step to evaluating our true past medical history is to know what big injuries we have to work with. Notice that I did not say "ignore." It's important to know what medical challenges we need to face. We will worry about how to overcome those challenges later in this book.

2. **Identify your stressors above the neck.**

This step is often ignored by unsuccessful athletes, young and old. It's extremely important to recognize your fears, anxieties, and motivators when upgrading your lifestyle. Being brave does not mean you're not scared. Being brave means even when you are scared, you still find a way to accomplish the scary feat. I recently overcame my fear of roller coasters by "wing walking" on the top wing of an acrobatic airplane.

3. **Identify your stressors below the neck.**

   Where are your common aches and pains located? Identifying them will help you treat those stressors. Let's say you have a common nagging pain in your lower back. The pain chips away at your morale and your positive attitude. Close your eyes and imagine using a few of the roller treatment tricks in this book to completely eliminate that pain. Now, being pain-free, think and feel how your attitude, mood, and posture will improve instantly!

4. **Know what the experts think.**

   I love to empower people to take control of their body and their health. But I never want people to ignore the valuable advice from healthcare experts they've consulted with in the past, and future. With this step, I want you to review your medical file and your memory for advice and tips shared by your healthcare team. Don't let that advice go unused or unappreciated. All that wellness insight may now prove especially helpful as you build your new body maintenance plan.

5. **Identify what your heart and head dream of doing.**

   Here's the fun part. Reflect back on what got you excited and motivated in the past. Do those dreams and visions make your heart quicken in a good way? Does the old vision of running the hometown 10-kilometer race still make you smile? Now merge your old dreams with your new dreams. Close your eyes, rid your mind of any *what if*s or *I can't do that*s, and just dream BIG!

TIP

Properly interpreting your true past medical history comes down to evaluating the three key elements that made you who you are over the past X number of years:

>> How I moved

>> What got me excited and what made me scared

>> What the medical experts thought about my body and mind

Body Assessment

Once you have a clear picture of your past medical history, it's time to turn your attention to your body. Before you plan your roller treatments, you need to take a thorough look at your own body to see where you need to focus some love.

REMEMBER

There is no such thing as the "perfect" body. Hollywood and social media will try to tell you differently, but it's not true. Understanding that point is necessary as you start to look at your own body in this chapter. When you look in the mirror or post pictures of yourself on your smartphone, you may not be excited about what you see. Relax. Breathe. Love the body and the person looking back at you.

This is a process of evaluating how your body moves today, improving how it will move tomorrow, and then repeating.

Some of this body assessment information involves details found in Chapter 11. I suggest reviewing that chapter for more details related to improving your posture in both standing and sitting.

Standing

Taking a deep dive into standing can help you improve your standing posture. My assessment model has proved to be very effective for improving the posture of individuals, young and old, for standing, walking, and squatting. The four components are as follows:

>> Describe what perfect posture looks like.

>> Body landmarks for perfect posture.

>> Positive signs for perfect posture.

>> Warning signs Blinking red lights (warning signs) for standing for bad posture.

Check out the following sections to apply this model for standing.

How someone describes seeing perfect standing

The following statements might be used to describe seeing someone in a perfect standing position:

"They're well balanced and tall."

"Their body just seems strong but relaxed."

"They don't seem to be working hard to just stand like that for hours."

Perfect standing posture

Perfect standing posture included the following components:

>> Your eyes are level with the floor, as seen in Figure 15-1a.

>> Your chin is comfortably positioned over the ribs.

>> Your shoulders are drawn back and down with little effort, as seen in Figure 15-1c.

>> Your chest is strong and positioned forward in a posture of power.

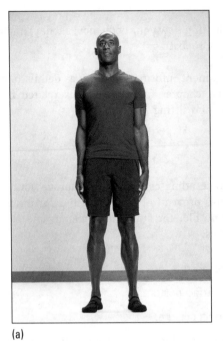

(a)

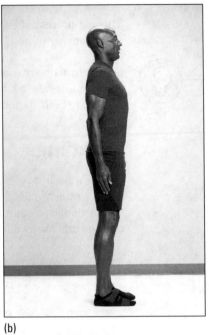

(b)

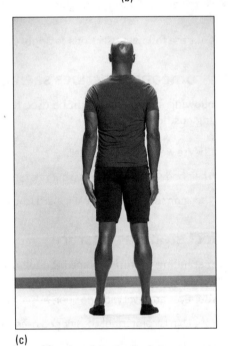

(c)

FIGURE 15-1:
Assessing
your standing
posture.

Photography by Haim Ariav and Klara Cu

>> Your arms rest beside the hips, hanging naturally from well-positioned shoulders.

>> The front of your pelvis is pulled upward, with strong lower abdominal muscles and flexible hip flexors, as seen in Figure 15-1b.

>> Your knees are slightly bent with strong, engaged quad muscles.

>> Your feet are strong and supportive, with or without shoes.

Positive signs to look for when standing

When you're standing with perfect posture, here is what you will see:

>> **Head is balanced.** The front of your chin is over your ribs at rest.

>> **Shoulders are in a position of power.** The shoulder blades are positioned back and low and within four inches of each other at rest.

>> **Spine is happy.** Looking from the side, the lower back has a mild sway, the upper back has a mild forward arch, and the neck has a mild sway.

>> **Bilateral symmetry.** One side of the body is positioned exactly the same as the other side.

>> **Level pelvis.** The pelvis is not overly tilted forward, and abdominal muscles are engaged.

>> **Base of support is well aligned.** Looking at the legs from the front, you can draw a straight line from the front of the hip to the front of the ankle.

>> **Busy toes.** The toes are engaged.

Blinking red lights (warning signs) for standing

Following are some warning signs to look for when your standing posture is poor and in need of correcting:

>> Winging shoulder blades when the insides of the shoulder blades pull away from the back of the ribs and point backwards.

>> Knocked knees, when the insides of the knees fall inward.

>> Clawed or pulled-back toes.

>> Forward head where the front of the chin is protruding well in front of the ribs.

>> Relaxed abdominals with a forward, rolled pelvis.

>> Rounded shoulders.

Walking

Walking is an activity most of us take for granted. We just do it with little thought on how we do it. Therefore, it's easy to get lazy when you walk. So it's easy to walk with terrible habits and poor posture. Don't let that happen because poor walking posture usually results in poor running posture.

How someone describes seeing perfect walking

The following statements may be used to describe seeing someone with perfect walking posture:

"They seem to just flow down the hall, almost effortlessly."

"Their body is well balanced, from one side to the other."

"It looks like no single joint is working too hard, and their hips, knees, and ankles all seem to move in perfect order."

Perfect walking posture

Perfect walking posture included the following components:

>> Your eyes are level with the floor, as seen in Figure 15-2a.

>> Your chin is comfortably positioned over the ribs.

>> One shoulder smoothly glides backwards as the opposite shoulder glides forward, and they appear to rotate around your navel.

>> Your chest stays high and strong.

>> Your arms swing comfortably like pendulums, hanging naturally from your symmetrically gliding shoulders, as seen in Figure 15-2b.

>> There is minimal space between your elbows and ribs, while your wrist teases the lateral thighs with symmetrical swings, as seen in Figure 15-2c.

>> The front of your pelvis stays high, with strong lower-abdominal muscles.

>> Your knees extend completely when pushing off and bend quickly as they swing forward.

>> Your ankle shows a large range of motion between being flat on the ground and pushing off.

>> Your feet are strong and supportive, with or without shoes.

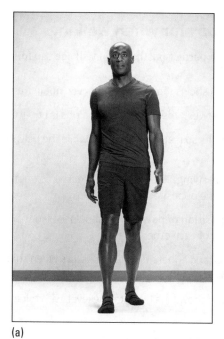

(a)

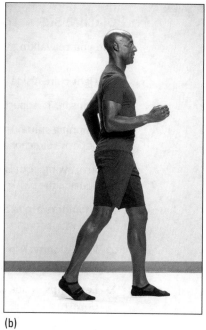

(b)

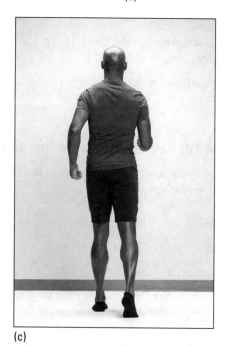

(c)

Photography by Haim Ariav and Klara Cu

FIGURE 15-2: Assessing your walking posture.

Positive signs to look for when walking

When you're walking with perfect posture, you will see the following:

- » **Tight chin.** A side view shows the head staying *over*, not in *front* of, the ribs.

- » **Arms in.** The space between the elbows and the ribs is equal on both sides.

- » **Spinning spine.** The ribs spin above the pelvis, while the pelvis spins in the opposite direction.

- » **Arm swing equals leg swing.** The amount of arm swing is approximately equal to the swing of the opposite leg.

- » **Shoulders are in a position of power.** The shoulder blades are back and low, and within four inches of each other at rest.

- » **Walk skinny.** Minimal and equal side-shifting occurs when shifting body weight from one foot to the other.

- » **Level hips.** A side view shows the hips staying level, with minimal up and down movement.

- » **Active cheeks.** A hind view shows both butt cheeks (glute muscles) contracting equally as strong.

- » **Bilateral symmetry.** One side of the body is doing the same as the other side.

- » **Equal feet.** Walking footprints in grass sand, or on a pool deck, are symmetrical.

Blinking red lights (warning signs) for walking

Following are some warning signs to look for when your walking posture is poor and in need of correcting:

- » Asymmetrical or uneven shoe-wear pattern on the bottom of your shoes

- » One leg is longer than the other

- » Uneven arm swing

- » Limited range of motion in a hip, knee, or ankle

- » Pain with walking

- » One leg shifts outward (circumduction) as it swings forward, more than the other leg

Squatting

We're all squatters. We squat in and out of a chair. We squat bending down to pick something off the floor. Squatting demands good lower extremity joint range of motion and muscle strength. Plan on becoming a stronger and more balanced squatter. When you do, squatting becomes a great way keep your hips and knee mobile while making your quads and glutes strong.

How someone describes seeing perfect squatting

The following statements might be used to describe seeing someone with perfect squatting form:

"They sure have loose, strong hips."

"Their spine stays so vertical, even when their hips drop low."

"They seem to drop straight down, thanks to really mobile ankles and flexible knees."

Perfect squatting posture

Perfect squatting form includes the following components:

>> You start with equal weight on both feet, with a tall, balanced posture, and with your hands comfortably holding a dowel level above your head, as seen in Figure 15-3a.

>> As you start your squat, your chest stays high, your shoulders stay back, your knees drift forward, and your heels stay flat on the ground.

>> At the bottom of the squat, your hands remain high and level, your shoulders are behind your knees, your thighs are level with the ground, and your weight is equal on both feet. See Figure 15-3b.

Positive signs to look for when squatting

When you're squatting with perfect form, this is what you will see:

>> **Loose and limber.** Hips, knees, and ankles all seem to move in equal proportion.

>> **High hands.** When squatting with a wooden dowel held overhead, the arms and dowel remain high at both the top and the bottom of the squat.

>> **Anchored heels.** The heels remain in contact with the ground from start to finish, as seen in Figure 15-3b.

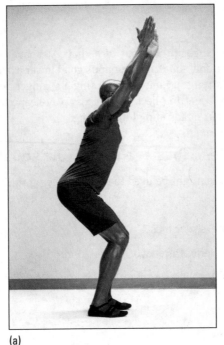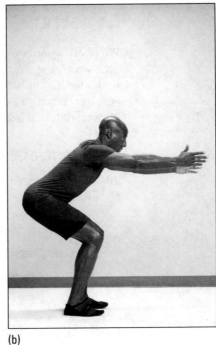

FIGURE 15-3:
Assessing your
squatting form. (a)   (b)

Photography by Haim Ariav and Klara Cu

>> **Sliding down the chimney chute.** The squatting motion appears vertical, strong, and fluid from start to finish.

>> **Strong hips.** The virtual axis of motion and power appears to come from the hips.

>> **Bilateral symmetry.** One side of the body is doing the same as the other side.

Blinking red lights (warning signs) for squatting

Here are the warning signs to look for when your squatting form is poor and in need of correcting:

>> A side view shows the shoulders quickly shifting forward in front of the knees when starting the squat.

>> A side view shows the elevated hands quickly shifting forward well in front of the shoulders, as seen in Figure 15-3c.

>> Pain with squatting.

>> A side view shows the spine is straight from the pelvis to the head.

>> A front view shows the body shifts to one side.

>> The heels raise off the ground when starting the squat.

Finding the Source of Your Pain

We get aches and pains, that's life. With our active lifestyle and our demanding jobs and sports, our bodies get pushed to their limits. My purpose in writing this book is to help you quickly manage those aches and pains to avoid them from becoming a limiting injury.

PT NOTE

One of my advantages, as a physical therapist, to staying active and healthy for so long is my ability to find the source of my aches and pains. Knowing the source of my pain allows me to properly treat the source. For example, if I determine the source of my calf tightness is coming from my fascia, I treat it very differently than if my tightness is coming from my calf muscles.

If you want to stay very active and reduce your risk of a serious injury, you need to learn how to separate the *source* of the pain from the *symptom* of the pain.

TIP

Think of it this way: What would you do if you found a puddle of water (the symptom) next to the wall in your living room from a hole in a water pipe (the source) located in the wall? Would you simply mop up the water (the symptom)? Or would you focus on finding the hole in the pipe (the source)?

I think we both know the answer to that question. If you first fix the source (your injury) of the puddle, getting rid of the puddle (your pain) is easy. Too often, I have patients and clients who come to me after spending too much time and too much money battling their symptoms (the puddle) while never truly addressing the source of those symptoms. In other words, they're spending too much of their valuable time mopping up their puddles.

I won't let this happen to you.

What a muscle injury feels like

OUCH

To better understand how to avoid injuries, it helps to better understand each injury. It's kind of a "know thy enemy," approach. To start your insightful sports medicine journey, consider what it feels like to have a muscle injury. When someone strains a muscle, this is what they feel:

>> If the injury happened suddenly when using the muscle, you felt the muscle fibers "pop."

>> The pain is very localized and intense.

>> Often you may assume, or hope, the injury is only a cramp. But unlike a cramp, a tearing of the muscle fibers, also called a *strain,* results in localized pain in an area typically smaller than a dollar bill.

>> The muscle seems to have a mind of its own, resulting in a protective spasm, or a "grab."

>> The area at and below the injury site becomes warm, swollen, and discolored with bleeding and bruising.

>> Over the next two to five days, when the injured muscle is stretched, a protective cramp is felt above and below the injury site.

What a joint injury feels like

OUCH

When someone sprains a joint, this is what they feel:

>> If the injury happens suddenly when you are using the muscle, you may feel a "pop," a shifting of the joint, or both.

>> The pain is instant.

>> Depending upon what part of the joint is injured, the location of the pain is either localized or deep inside the joint where you "just can't put your finger right on it."

>> The joint range of motion is instantly reduced.

>> The active movement of the joint "just feels different," like something has changed inside the joint.

>> The type of pain can vary greatly because of the many different types of joint tissues involved. The types of pain include catching, stabbing, aching, sharp, or shifting.

>> If the joint is in the lower extremity, the pain increases with weight bearing while the joint may instantly feel unstable. Typically, the faster you walk or run, the worse the symptoms become.

>> Depending upon the severity of the injury and the type of tissue (bone, articular cartilage, capsule, fibrocartilage, fascia, or ligament), the swelling can be mild or severe.

>> The location of most of the swelling is inside the joint capsule.

What a bone injury feels like

OUCH

When someone fractures a bone, this is what they feel:

>> When a bone breaks, you know it.

>> The location of the pain is very isolated and intense.

- Unless the bone injury is deep within a joint, you can usually put one finger on the exact location of the injury.

- A deep aching inside the bone is a common symptom because bones are so important to stabilizing and protecting the body.

- Even mild motion or weight bearing on an injured bone increases the pain.

- My early childhood playground rule, "If you can move it, it's not broken," is a big lie!! (To my childhood friends with whom I used this flawed diagnostic protocol I'm sorry.)

- Immediate medical care is needed to avoid worsening the serious bone injury.

- There are other types of bone injuries besides simple fractures.

OUCH

What a nerve injury feels like

When someone injures a nerve, this is what they experience:

- I just have to say it right up front: Nerve injuries can be strange and unusual.

- Case in point: A nerve injury can produce symptoms involving burning, numbness, aching, pins-and-needles, shooting, tingling, and weakness. That's a wide range of symptoms!

- Nerve injuries can happen quickly or slowly.

- The location of the symptoms can be far away from the nerve injury. An example of this is when you injure your "funny bone" on the back inside of your elbow. Although the injury is at your elbow, most of the symptoms are felt 15 to 18 inches away, in your pinky and ring finger.

- Mild nerve injuries typically produce mild changes in sensation, including numbness.

- More severe nerve injuries produce more severe symptoms, including muscle weakness.

- Nerve injuries can resolve quickly or slowly.

OUCH

What overly tight fascia feel like

When someone's fascia is too tight, this is what they feel:

- Fascia-related injuries can test your patience because they have a wide range of causes, symptoms, and solutions.

- » Fascia injuries can happen quickly or slowly.

- » The pain is usually not sharp or overly intense.

- » The symptoms are typically more generalized, and include pressure, tightness, and aching.

- » The injury is usually not very localized but occurs over a slightly larger area, depending on the body part.

- » The symptoms may improve or worsen with motion and exercise involving the body part.

- » When you're feeling the area involving the overly tight fascia, the area feels more bounded down and rigid, compared to the other side.

- » The tissue in the area of the fascia lesion does not feel swollen, but it may feel overly warm.

Putting Your Scouting Report Together

Wow, that's a lot of injury information to think about. I wouldn't blame you if you needed to take a breather, get a drink of cold water, and give yourself a few minutes to let your brain marinate in all this sports medicine info.

(Pause here and again review the body-scouting information most pertinent to you. This is all about *you* gaining control of your body and your injuries.)

Welcome back!

Okay, so let's learn how you can use this information in a simple way to help you prevent injuries, manage your present body issues, and stay pain-free.

REMEMBER

Here's what you did in this chapter:

- » You reviewed your true past medical history.

- » You evaluated how you stand.

- » You evaluated how you walk.

- » You evaluated how you squat.

- » You learned the true value of treating the *source* of your pain instead of the *symptom* of your pain.

- » You took a deep look at how different tissues feel when they become injured to better understand the source of your pain.

Now it's time to pull all this valuable information together. Granted, you have a significant amount of information to comprehend. But the value of understanding how you are presently moving is very important to help you achieve your goal of moving with a greater range of motion and less pain.

Evaluating your TPMH

What body part is your "Achilles heel" or weak spot? As you review your thorough medical history involving your activities, mindsets, and healthcare provider information, look for commonalities. Most of them may be very obvious; for example, maybe you had a couple of knee surgeries after an old knee injury.

But some of the sources of your past injuries may not be so obvious. This means it's time for you to play detective. Take a moment to step back and look at your entire body, knowing your medical history. Are there any patterns or trends that you may have overlooked? You may find most of your past injuries and pain involve only one side of your body.

You may reflect back upon advice that a healthcare provider gave you in the past, which you forgot about. As you look back at patterns that have both helped and hurt you, they will provide you with helpful information going forward.

Identifying blinking red lights (warning signs)

Having the opportunity, with smartphone pictures and videos, to look at yourself standing, walking, and squatting has given you priceless information. You may have been surprised or even shocked to watch how you move. It's a much different view of yourself compared to those pretty selfies you take with your friends.

TIP

I want you to compare what you saw in your self-photos and videos with the photos and perfect-posture information you read earlier in this chapter. Also, reviewing the posture photos and information in Chapter 11 will be helpful as you assess your body postures.

TIP

With that comparison, I want you to find your blinking red lights. By that, I mean I want you to identify your problem areas. Identifying these areas helps you to identify the source of your pain. Even though the blinking red lights may cause major changes in the way you move, many times the solution to fix these problems can be quite simple.

Here are some examples of common blinking red lights found in standing, walking, and squatting assessments:

>> Poor posture

>> Forward head

>> Poor balance

>> Stiff spine

>> Rounded shoulders

>> Tight hips

>> Stiff knees

>> Weak abs

>> Tight calves or ankles

>> Pronated feet

Identifying these problem areas will help you properly treat the injury with a roller.

Matching blinking red lights with tissue symptoms

Now you know which body parts have had previous problems and which body parts are not moving properly. Some of those past injuries and present moving issues are perfect matches. Meanwhile, some of the new moving problems may simply be the result of you compensating for old injuries.

If you broke your foot five years ago and it forced you to limp for three months, there's a pretty good chance you may still have some of that limp when you walk but not know it. As you learned a few chapters ago, your brain and body are very good at compensating around an injury. So, often, when the injury has healed, the brain has not been given a reason to discontinue the compensation, and that new movement pattern becomes the norm.

The information in this chapter is very effective in helping you clean up, so to speak, the way you move. If your car has one wheel out of alignment, the entire car is affected. The longer you drive your car with poor wheel alignment involving only one wheel, or 25 percent of the wheelbase, the more damage you are doing to the other three wheels, brakes, struts, steering, and frame.

Your body is no different. It's time for you to get a wheel alignment.

TIP

Okay, Detective, it's time to wrap up your case. Let's put your body scouting report together:

1. List your blinking red lights, or troubled body parts.

2. With each blinking red light, list the symptoms you have felt in that body part in the last two months.

3. Compare the list of symptoms with the "What an X injury feels like" section.

4. Start to determine what types of tissues in certain body parts seem to be obvious troublemakers, or the source of your pain.

Well done, Detective! Now you have visual evidence of the crime scenes (troubled body parts) *and* a list of the probable suspects (painful tissues). *That's* valuable information as you get closer to making pain a thing of the past!

Chapter **16**

Unlocking Your Upper Legs

When muscles are tight and bound down, your body has to work harder just to move. Imagine how hard you would need to work walking up three flights of stairs wearing wet, tight jeans. This too-small-skinny-jean syndrome is exactly what happens when your thigh muscles are tight and restrictive. As I discuss in Chapter 8, your body will move faster and with less effort when your muscles, tendons, and fascia are relaxed and elastic.

PT NOTE

Improving the elastic nature of a muscle can take place faster and last longer when you properly roll the muscle compared to when you simply stretch it. With a roller and the treatments in this book, you can quickly relax, or as I like to say, "unlock" tight muscles and their surrounding fascia. The proper term I like to use for treating tight muscle and fascia is *self-myofascial unlocking*.

In this chapter, I cover techniques to relax or unlock your upper leg muscles, focusing on four different zones:

» Front of thigh, quads

» Outside of thigh, iliotibial band

>> Inside of thigh, groin

>> Back of thigh, hamstrings

TIP

Don't think of a roller as a painful weapon to "beat-up" your muscles. Instead, think of your roller as a tool to "unlock" your valuable muscles. Kicking in a locked door takes power and hard work. Meanwhile, unlocking the same door with a key is much easier and faster. In this chapter, I want to show you the right "keys" to unlock the muscles of your upper leg.

Ryan Rolling Rules for the Upper Legs

REMEMBER

Take a few minutes to look back over Chapter 8 to review my five rolling rules. These rules explain the simple roller-treatment steps you follow to roll your muscles safely and effectively. The order of these steps is important.

1. Align the spine.

Proper posture on the roller is the first step, and also your first priority. It's a simple way to protect the spine as you unlock upper leg muscles, eliminate trigger points, and relax tight fascia on the roller or roller ball.

2. Breathe.

Don't hold your breath while rolling. Poor breathing habits make your body tighten up and go into a protective state. When that happens, your benefits from rolling are drastically reduced. You don't want that. Roller Breathing 101 states, "inhale and exhale slowly, deeply, and loudly."

3. Slow roll.

Give your body more time for positive changes to occur. You can accomplish this by moving slowly on the roller. The roller techniques for the tight upper leg muscles requires a slow roller speed.

4. Seek and destroy.

It's hunting season, so go hunt for painful trigger points in the muscles of your upper leg. Trigger points and adhesions make your muscles weak and your joints tight. Use your roller to seek and destroy those ugly trigger points.

5. Move the muscle.

Level 2 treatments add movement to your roller treatments. When active movement is added to your treatment, the entire muscle from tendon to tendon and its fascia are lengthened through a larger range of motion.

Unlocking the Quads (aka the Workhorses)

The four power muscles on the front side of the thigh are called the quadriceps muscles, or quads for short (see Figure 16-1). These four muscles run the length of the femur or thigh bone, and anchor on the top of the patella or kneecap. Together, the quads are often referred to as the "workhorses" of the leg.

PT NOTE

Three of the quad muscles attach on the upper thigh bone. The fourth muscle, the mighty rectus femoris, is the only quad muscle that crosses the hip joint. Because it's the longest quad muscle and, with the help of the kneecap and patella tendon, the only quad muscle to cross both the knee and hip joints, the busy rectus femoris is usually the tightest quad muscle and will therefore be the focus of your roller treatments.

If you're pulling an expensive boat through a narrow canal, you'll have much more control using four medium-size ropes attached to the boat compared to using only one big rope attached to your treasured yacht. Applying this analogy to your thigh, if your four quad muscles are tight and bound together, they'll pull on your kneecap and knee joint like one big, tight muscle instead of four independent, strong, and mobile muscles.

This unlocking treatment will relax the four quad muscles and a smaller, less important quad-wannabe muscle. By unlocking your quad muscles, this treatment allows all four muscles to do their specific jobs independently. These are strong muscles responsible for straightening your knee joint and lifting the leg forward at the hip joint — two important movements for walking and running.

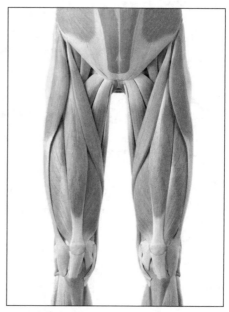

SciePro/Shutterstock

FIGURE 16-1:
The workhorses' stable located on the front of the thigh.

Getting ready

Lay face down towards the top half of your padded launch pad. Place the roller just above the kneecap, perpendicular to the leg. Rest comfortably on both elbows in a plank-like position. Swing the other knee outward, placing some of your weight on the inside of your bent knee.

If this starting position is uncomfortable for your knees or elbows, use pillows or towels to support your body weight.

As you prepare to unlock or relax tight muscles, now is a good time to start your slow and deep breathing pattern.

TIP

Before you start any rolling treatment or exercise, it helps to quiet your body and mind. Close your eyes. Visualize your body resting in a relaxed and pain-free place. Perform three slow, deep breaths to prepare your body to heal.

The exercise

Here's how you can relax your quad muscles by unlocking their trigger points.

1. **Start by slowly rolling your leg downward, which allows the roller to glide upwards towards the hip, as shown in Figure 16-2.**

    Moving your elbows and bent knee downward, slowly run the roller up the front of the thigh, searching for trigger points or areas of tightness. I playfully refer to these localized muscle restrictions with my physical therapy patients as "painful grapes." Your job is to find all the painful grapes on the front side of the thigh and crush them.

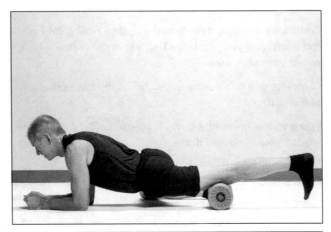

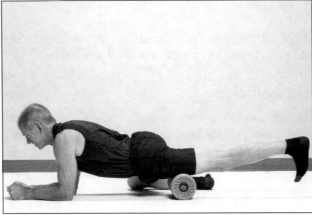

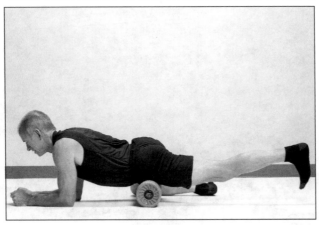

FIGURE 16-2:
Rolling the quad muscles — starting, middle, and finishing positions.

Photography by Haim Ariav and Klara Cu

2. Continue with loud, deep breathing, slow rolling, and grape crushing up the thigh until you reach the finish line: the crease where your thigh meets your abdomen.

3. Complete one roll in an upward direction; it will take approximately one minute.

4. When you've finished, safely lift yourself off the roller and pat yourself on the back for a job well done.

Level 1 unlocking

Rest on each painful grape for three slow breaths, allowing the roller to melt into the muscle like a hot knife through butter. Then resume the upward roll, seeking more trigger points.

If your quads are both looser and pain-free with walking after a minimum of three days of Level 1 unlocking, progress to Level 2 unlocking.

Level 2 unlocking

Rest on each painful grape for three slow breaths, allowing the roller to melt into the muscle. Next, slowly bend the knee approximately 45 degrees before slowly returning to the straight position, as shown in Figure 16-3. Perform this slow bend two times in each direction on each trigger point.

FIGURE 16-3:
Level 2 quad treatments involve adding a slow, 45-degree knee bend, then returning to a straight knee position two times on each trigger point.

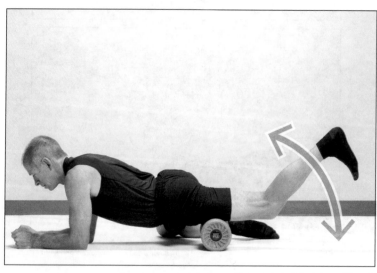

Photography by Haim Ariav and Klara Cu

Note how much the muscle-unlocking intensity increases when knee motion is added.

Resume your seek-and-destroy mission up the front of your thigh, looking for the next painful grape.

WARNING

Bending the knee too far during Level 2 quad treatments can trigger a painful hamstring spasm. Been there, done that. Those of us who carelessly bent our knees past 45 degrees while rolling our quads and then suffered the wrath of three angry hamstring muscles in full spasms only made that mistake once! I hope you learn from my painful mistake.

Do's and don'ts

Keep the following do's and don'ts in mind when rolling the muscles in the front of your thigh:

>> Do breathe slow, deep, and loud.

>> Do move the roller in one direction: upward towards the hip.

>> Do try other roller options, like vibrating rollers and roller balls, to determine the best options to unlock your quad muscles.

>> Do use towels, pillows, or pads to keep weight-bearing body parts like your elbows happy.

COMMON SOURCES OF KNEE PAIN INVOLVING LEG MUSCLES

Dysfunctional leg muscles and knee pain go hand-in-hand. If your quads are weak, your knees are overloaded every time your feet hit the ground. If your leg muscles are too tight, your knees are over-compressed every time you bend your knees.

- Weak quad muscle

- Tight hamstrings

- Adhesions on distal iliotibial band

- Tight rectus femorus quad muscle

- Strength imbalance between quads and hamstrings at fast contraction speeds

>> Don't roll on your kneecap or hip bone.

>> Don't roll on an acutely strained quad muscle.

>> Don't roll on any area that produces numbness, tingling, shooting pain, or weakness.

Unlocking your Iliotibial Band (ITB)

A common source of lateral knee pain and tight legs is the lateral side of the thigh. A short, strong muscle with a busy name, the *tensor fascia lata* (TFL) starts on the outside of your pelvis just below the beltline. The TFL quickly merges with a long, strong band called the *iliotibial band* or ITB. The ITB runs all the way down the outside of the thigh, anchoring to the larger shin bone just below the knee, as shown in Figure 16-4.

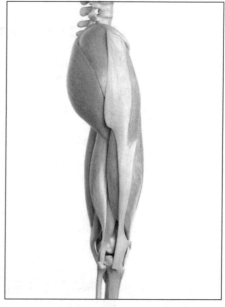

SciePro/Shutterstock

PT NOTE

One of the reasons why this short muscle belly/long tendon band is such a troublemaker is that it lays right on top of the largest of the quad muscles. Without consistent rolling and stretching, the quads' vastus lateralis muscle engulfs the skinny ITB. When this happens, the ITB typically becomes tight and painful on the outside of the knee and along the distal thigh.

FIGURE 16-4:
The short, strong TFL muscle feeds into the ITB as it lays firmly on top of the quads' vastus lateralis muscle.

Fear not, your roller rescue is here to keep you pain-free!

TIP

When rolling the outside of the thigh, remember the motto: "Stay straight from your head to your heel." This protects your lower back from injury and maximizes the results of your rolling treatment.

Getting ready

Position yourself in a side-plank position towards the bottom half of your padded launch pad. Place the roller just below your lateral beltline, perpendicular to your spine. Rest comfortably on your elbow with your upper leg's foot placed on the pad in front of your lower thigh.

To help you to stay straight from your head to your heel, continue to point your upper hand towards the sky while you look straight ahead, keeping your head in line with your spine.

OUCH

If this starting position is uncomfortable for your elbow, use pillows or pads to provide extra padding under your bent elbow.

As you prepare to unlock or relax tight muscles, now is a good time to start your slow and deep breathing pattern.

TIP

Before you start any rolling treatment or exercise, it helps to quiet your body and mind. Close your eyes. Visualize your body resting in a relaxed and pain-free place. Perform three slow, deep breaths to prepare your body to heal.

The exercise

Here's how to relax your lateral thigh by unlocking its trigger points.

PT NOTE

1. **Start by slowly rolling your leg upward, which conversely allows the roller to move downwards towards the knee, as shown in Figure 16-5.**

   By moving your bent elbow and foot upward, slowly glide the roller down the outside of the thigh, searching for those tender trigger points. With slow rolling and continuous deep breathing, find the painful grapes down the lateral thigh and crush them.

2. **Continue with loud, deep breathing, slow rolling, and painful grape-crushing down the lateral thigh until you reach the finish line: the bony ridge on the outside of the knee.**

3. **Complete one roll in a downward direction; it will take approximately one minute.**

   When you're done, safely lift yourself off the roller by rolling forward into a face-down position.

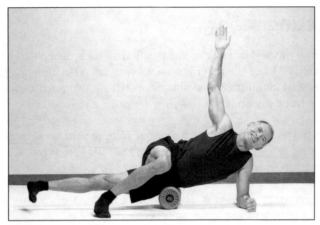

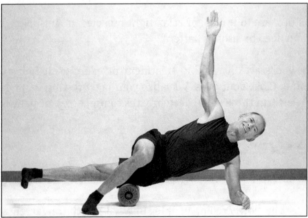

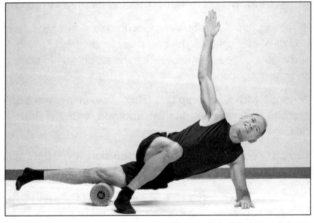

FIGURE 16-5: Rolling your ITB and lateral thigh — starting, middle, and ending positions.

Photography by Haim Ariav and Klara Cu

Level 1 unlocking

Rest on each trigger point for three slow breaths, allowing the roller to melt into the muscle like a hot knife through butter. Then resume the downward roll, seeking the next painful grape.

If your ITB is looser and pain-free with walking after a minimum of three days of Level 1 unlocking, progress to Level 2 unlocking.

OUCH

If you think Level 1 ITB treatments hurt, wait until you hit Level 2! Tread slowly on this one.

Level 2 unlocking

Rest on each painful grape for three slow breaths, allowing the roller to melt into the muscle. Next, slowly bend the rolling knee to approximately 45 degrees before slowly returning to the straight-knee position (see Figure 16-6). Perform this slow bend two times in each direction on each trigger point.

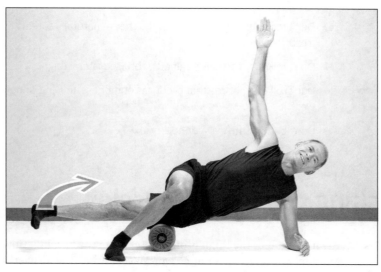

FIGURE 16-6:
Level 2 ITB treatments involve adding a slow, 45-degree knee bend.

Photography by Haim Ariav and Klara Cu

Note how much the muscle unlocking–intensity increases when knee motion is added.

Resume your seek-and-destroy mission down the side of your thigh, looking for the next painful grape.

OUCH

When you are rolling the lower ITB, it can be quite tender and uncomfortable. Maintain your stellar alignment, keep breathing, and kiss those annoying trigger points good-bye!

Do's and don'ts

Ask any serious runners you know and they will tell you: ITB pain is a nightmare. Here are some do's and don'ts to help you properly unlock your ITB and lateral thigh muscles.

>> Do stay straight from your "head to your heel" by keeping your upper hand pointing straight skyward, your head in line with your spine, and your hips forward.

>> Do breathe slow, deep, and loud.

>> Do move the roller in one direction: downward towards the knee.

>> Do try other roller options, like vibrating rollers and roller balls, to determine the best ways to unlock your lateral thigh muscles.

>> Don't roll your ITB too aggressively. They're naturally sore without Level 2 treatment movement.

>> Don't roll on an acutely strained or bruised lateral thigh.

>> Don't roll on any area that produces numbness, tingling, shooting pain, or weakness.

>> Don't bend at the waist or neck.

Unlocking the Groin Muscles

PT NOTE

The inner half of the thigh is often referred to the "groin". How many muscles do you think make up the groin? Two? Maybe three? The answer is six! And in addition to those six very diverse groin muscles, this zone of the thigh also involves parts of quad muscles, hamstring muscles, hip-flexing muscles, and too many nerves and blood vessels to count. The bottom line is that your inner thigh, as shown in Figure 16-7, is a very busy and important part of your leg.

With that being said, keeping the muscles and fascia in your inner thigh unlocked is important if you want to be active and pain-free.

Before you start any rolling treatment or exercise, it helps to quiet your body and mind. Close your eyes. Visualize your body resting in a relaxed and pain-free place. Perform three slow, deep breaths to prepare your body to heal.

Getting ready

Lay face down in the middle of your padded launch pad. Keep one leg straight. Bend your other knee approximately 45 degrees. Place the roller on the upper, inner, flexed thigh, perpendicular to the leg. Rest comfortably on both elbows in a plank-like position.

If this starting position is uncomfortable for your elbows or knees, use pillows or pads to support your body weight.

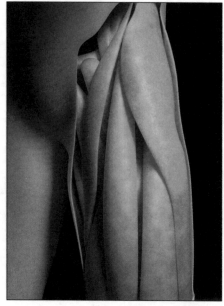

David Marchal/Shutterstock

FIGURE 16-7:
The busy and complicated landscape of the inside of the thigh.

As you prepare to unlock or relax tight muscles, now is a good time to start your slow and deep breathing pattern.

The exercise

Here's how you can relax your groin muscles by unlocking their trigger points.

1. **Start by slowly shifting your body upward away from the roller, as shown in Figure 16-8.**

   This will allow the roller to move down the inside of the flexed thigh, fishing for tender trigger points.

   Maintain deep breathing and a downward direction when slow rolling.

2. **Continue with loud, deep breathing, slow rolling down the inner thigh until you reach the finish line: the bony ridge on the inside of the knee.**

3. **Complete one roll in a downward direction; it will take approximately one minute.**

   When you're done, safely lift yourself off the roller by shifting your body weight to your other leg.

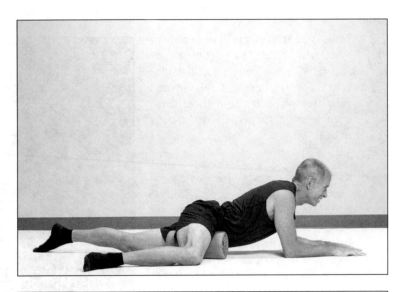

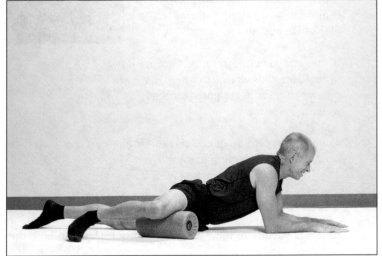

Photography by Haim Ariav and Klara Cu

Level 1 unlocking

Rest on each painful grape for three slow breaths, allowing the roller to melt into the muscle like a hot knife through butter. Then resume the downward roll, seeking more tender trigger points.

If your groin muscles are both looser and pain-free with walking after a minimum of three days of Level 1 unlocking, progress to Level 2 unlocking.

Level 2 unlocking

Rest on each painful grape for three slow breaths, allowing the roller to melt into the muscle. Next, slowly straighten the knee before slowly returning to a bent position (see Figure 16-9). Perform this slow extension movement two times in each direction on each trigger point. Then return to stomping on more painful grapes.

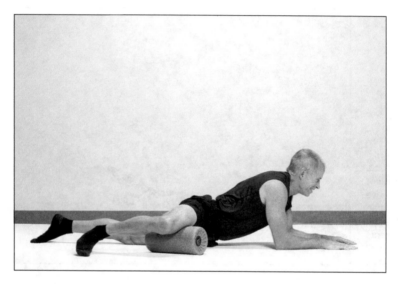

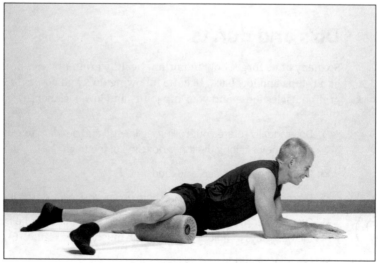

FIGURE 16-9: Level 2 groin treatments involve adding a slow knee extension.

Photography by Haim Ariav and Klara Cu

Note how much the muscle-unlocking intensity increases when knee motion is added.

TIP

To treat more isolated trigger points or adhesions in the inner thigh, use a small roller ball. Start with Level 1 by resting on the painful grapes, and then slowly progress to Level 2 treatments by adding active movements, as shown in Figure 16-10.

FIGURE 16-10:
A more aggressive game plan involves groin treatments with a small roller ball.

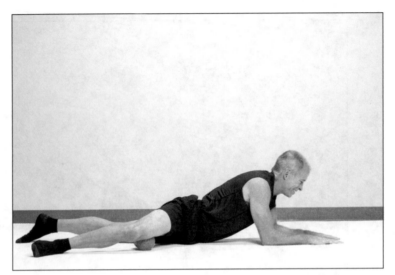

Photography by Haim Ariav and Klara Cu

Do's and don'ts

So many of us forget how important healthy groin muscles are for the well-being of our hips and low back. Use the following do's and don'ts to keep all six of your groin muscles loose and your hip joints and low back happy.

>> Do gradually rotate your rolling leg inward and outward to expose more trigger points along the inner ridgeline of the thigh.

>> Do breathe slow, deep, and loud.

>> Do move the roller in one direction: downward towards the inner knee.

TIP

>> Do try other roller options, like vibrating rollers and roller balls, to determine the best ways to unlock your six groin muscles (see Figure 16-11).

>> Do adjust your hip and pelvis positions to alter the roller treatments.

>> Don't roll your calf muscles too aggressively to avoid making your calf tighter.

>> Don't roll on swollen glands on the inner thigh.

>> Don't roll on any area that produces numbness, tingling, shooting pain, or weakness.

>> Don't start too high. I'll leave it at that.

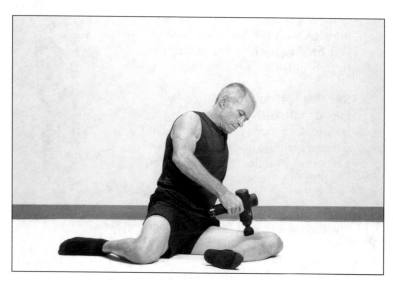

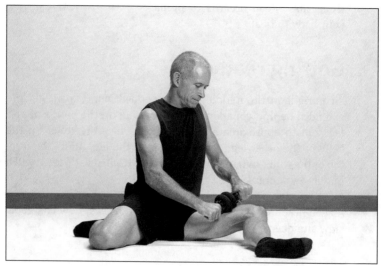

FIGURE 16-11: Manual groin treatment options.

Photography by Haim Ariav and Klara Cu

Unlocking the Hamstrings

The back of the thigh is the home for three muscles called the *hamstrings*, as shown in Figure 16-12. The three long muscles start on the backside of the pelvis, travel the entire length of the thigh, and anchor into the back of the upper shin bone. They're busy muscles, with the important task of both bending the knee and pulling the thigh bone backwards at the hip joint.

Knowing how much work the hammies do with each and every step you take *and* how much time you spend in a seated position, it's no surprise your hamstring muscles are often tight and inflexible.

TIP

Before you start any rolling treatment or exercise, it helps to quiet your body and mind. Close your eyes. Visualize your body resting in a relaxed and pain-free place. Perform three slow, deep breaths to prepare your body to heal.

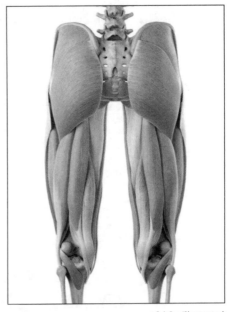

SciePro/Shutterstock

FIGURE 16-12:
The hammies — the three muscles on the backside of the thigh.

Getting ready

Sit upright in the middle of your padded launch pad. Recline backwards, arms extended behind you, comfortably resting on the palms of both hands. Keep one leg bent to approximately 90 degrees. Place the roller on the upper hamstring belly of the other leg, perpendicular to the leg. Allow the treated leg to relax on top of the roller. When you do this, your treated leg's knee will be bent to approximately 25 degrees.

As you prepare to unlock or relax tight muscles, now is a good time to start your slow and deep breathing pattern.

The exercise

Here's how you can relax your hamstring muscles by unlocking their trigger points.

1. **As shown in Figure 16-13, start by slowly shifting your body backwards like a crab, by pushing with the other leg and walking the hands backwards.**

    This motion allows the roller to move down the back of the thigh.

2. **By now you know the game plan: find painful grapes, crush painful grapes, repeat.**

    Maintain deep breathing and slow rolling downward.

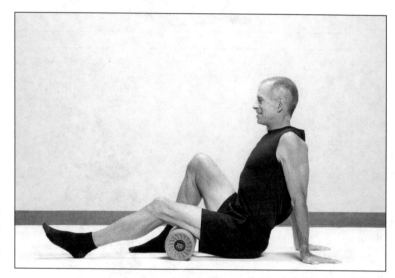

FIGURE 16-13:
Rolling the three hamstring muscles.

Photography by Haim Ariav and Klara Cu

TIP

When rolling the back of the thigh, try rotating your leg side to side, as shown in Figure 16-14. This will widen the healing path of your roller to treat the bellies of all three hamstring muscles.

3. **Continue down the back of the thigh until you reach the finish line: the upper belly of the calf muscles.**

4. **Complete one roll in a downward direction; it will take approximately one minute.**

    When you're done, roll yourself off the roller by shifting your body weight to your other leg.

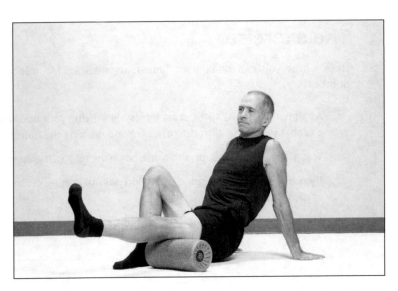

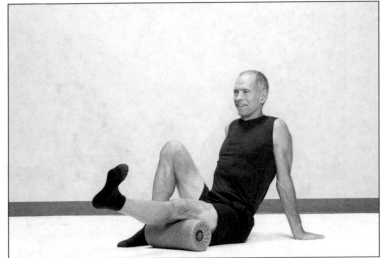

Photography by Haim Ariav and Klara Cu

FIGURE 16-14:
Rotating the
treated leg
will isolate the
inner or outer
hamstring
muscles.

Level 1 unlocking

Rest on each painful grape for three slow breaths, allowing the roller to melt into the muscle like a hot knife through butter. Then resume the downward roll, seeking additional tender trigger points.

If your hamstrings are both looser and pain-free with walking after a minimum of three days of Level 1 unlocking, progress to Level 2 unlocking.

Level 2 unlocking

Rest on each tender trigger point for three slow breaths, allowing the roller to melt into the muscle. Next, by tightening the quads, slowly straighten the bent knee, as shown in Figure 16-15, before slowly returning it to a bent position. Perform this slow extension movement two times in each direction on each trigger point. Then return to stomping on more painful grapes.

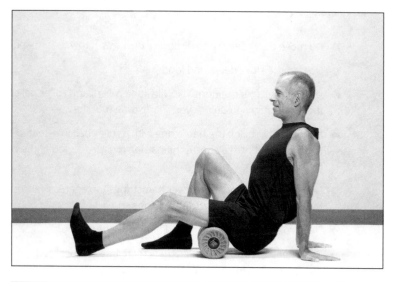

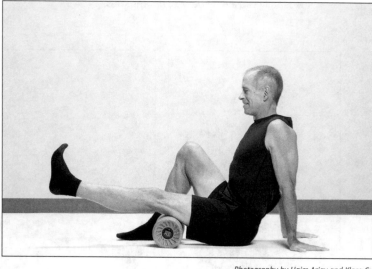

FIGURE 16-15:
Level 2 hamstring treatments involve adding a slow knee extension, then returning to a bent-knee position, two times on each trigger point.

Photography by Haim Ariav and Klara Cu

Note how much the muscle–unlocking intensity increases when knee motion is added.

Do's and don'ts

Here are a few tips to mastering the rolling techniques for your hamstring. They will help you unlock your hard-working "hammies" fast while avoiding common mistakes.

>> Do move the roller in one direction: downward towards the back of the knee.

>> Do breathe slow, deep, and loud.

>> Do try other roller options, like vibrating rollers and roller balls, to determine the best options to unlock your hamstring muscles.

>> Do play with rolling the hamstring with a roller ball in a seated position to start the treatment with a shorter hamstring muscle to modify the results (see Figure 16-16).

>> Don't roll your upper and lower hamstrings too aggressively to avoid making the upper or lower hamstring tendons sore.

>> Don't roll on an acutely strained hamstring muscle.

>> Don't keep pressure on spots that create intense localized burning, tingling, numbness, or pins-and-needles sensations down the leg. Those symptoms are usually caused by nerves, not muscles.

FIGURE 16-16:
Alternative Level 2 hamstring treatments in a chair with a roller ball. This figure shows the starting and finishing positions.

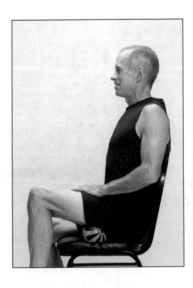
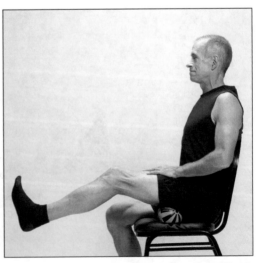

Photography by Haim Ariav and Klara Cu

Chapter **17**

Unlocking Your Lower Legs and Feet

I n Chapter 16, I refer to the quads as the "leg workhorses." I'm not backing off my praise of the big fellas upstairs, but I do want to show some love to the blue-collared grinders below the knees. The tough workers of the lower leg include strong calves in the back, stabilizing peroneals on the side, the anterior tibialis muscle up front, and dozens of muscles in the ankle and arch of the foot. These important groups of muscles, tendons, and fascia may not get much hype, but if you don't keep them healthy and happy, your social media–hungry quads will soon be sitting on the bench! Let's get to work.

The lower leg treatments in this chapter are divided into four zones:

» Calf

» Outside lower shin

» Front of shin

» Arch

PT NOTE

Kinesiology terminology: When the foot is pointed downward, as you would do when pushing on your car's gas pedal, that motion is referred to as *plantar flexion.* Conversely, when the foot is pulled upward towards the knee, it is referred to as *dorsiflexion.*

An Inside Look at the Lower Legs and Feet

This chapter focuses on unlocking your grinder muscles in the lower leg below the knee. Most of these muscles and tendons work hard within a limited range of motion. The normal limited range of motion makes the muscles and the fascia of the lower leg much tighter than the upper leg.

TIP

Step back and look at your legs in the mirror. You can easily see that each leg is much wider on the top and tapers or narrows as you move downward towards the foot (see Figure 17-1).

PT NOTE

It's time for a skin tension test. Pinch and pull on the skin around your thigh, as well as on your lower shin. Do you notice a difference? Unless you're wearing a scuba diving wet-suit, the skin on your shin is much tighter. Your shin skin is cinched down to the fascia, muscle, and bone just beneath the skin.

Following are a few of the design traits that make the lower leg highly prone to injury:

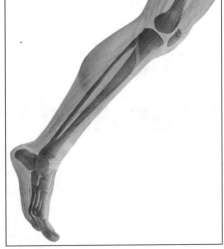

Adapted from adike/Shutterstock

FIGURE 17-1:
Lower leg in motion.

>> Muscles and tendons have a limited range of motion.

>> The anatomy is congested in a smaller area at the bottom of the leg.

>> Blood flow in the lower leg is restricted because your foot is literally a circulatory cul-de-sac.

>> The lymphatic system, the sewer system of the extremities, is forced to drain the leg muscles' waste products uphill, against gravity.

>> Fascial tissue is tighter in the lower leg.

>> The skin of the lower leg is tighter.

>> One hundred percent of your body weight rests on a relatively small surface area, equal to the approximate size of three one-dollar bills (see Figure 17-2).

The lower legs deserve more love because they do so much work to keep us active. Our feet are often referred to as the "dogs." I'm a big dog lover, so my feet love that expression. Witnessing the loyal and unconditional love my two rescue dogs at home show my family and me every day, I see the title of *dog* as a huge compliment.

Too often, we make life more difficult for our lower legs. That has to stop. We know how important our lower legs and feet are for our active life. Before you jump on the "Love Thy Feet" train, let's work on putting a halt to the things that hurt your lower legs and feet.

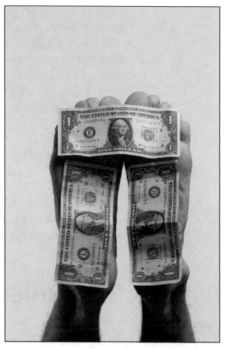

Photography by Haim Ariav & Klara Cu

FIGURE 17-2:
You balance your entire body on two tiny pieces of real estate equal to the size of three one-dollar bills.

OUCH

Following are things you do that hurt your lower legs and feet:

>> Gain weight

>> Wear tight shoes

>> Eat poorly

>> Stop walking barefoot, resulting in weaker feet and arches

>> Stop stretching your calves

>> Wear elevated (high) heel shoes

>> Stay inactive, thus reducing control of foot muscles (responsible for balance)

>> Sit too long, resulting in swollen ankles

>> Reduce your fitness level, resulting in weaker lower leg and core muscles

When you push off the foot, the last part of your body to leave the ground is the toes. Now take a look at all the toes around you. Take a gander at your toes, your kids' toes, the toes of your friends and family. The only thing you probably noticed is how different each of them are. Toes are the last point of contact for the complicated mechanical process of walking, running, and jumping. We see great toe function variations, even from side-to-side for the same person, as well as between different individuals.

With that being said, the manner in which each of us walks, runs, and jumps is also somewhat different. This variation, even from one leg to the other, puts an altered load on the muscles, tendons, and fascia of the lower leg.

PT NOTE

Here's where a roller and roller ball come to the rescue: Keeping your already bound-down and hard-working muscles, tendons, and fascia moving properly will quickly improve your movement patterns and reduce your pain.

Ryan Rolling Rules for Lower Legs and Feet

REMEMBER

Following are my five "rolling rules" to be used when you perform any treatment with a roller. I strongly suggest that you take a few minutes to review the details of these five rules back in Chapter 8. They will help you roll safely and be much more effective with your roller treatments.

1. Align the spine.

This is another way of using proper posture on the roller. As you change body positions on the roller to unlock lower leg muscles, eliminate trigger points, and relax tight fascia, it's still a high priority to protect your spine.

2. Breathe.

If you hold your breath while rolling, which is a natural response when in pain, the outcome of your roller treatments will suffer. Stated bluntly, if you're a bad breather, you'll be a bad roller. Being a good breather is easy: Inhale and exhale slowly, deeply, and loudly.

3. Slow roll.

The roller techniques for the tight tissue of the lower leg and foot require a slow roller speed. A slower-moving roller allows the body the more time to make positive changes.

4. Seek and destroy.

It's time to go hunting. You've been given a lifetime trigger-point hunting license. You have plenty of painful trigger points scattered throughout your body, making your muscles and joints tighter than they're supposed to be. Trigger points also make your muscles weak. Seeking and destroying trigger points with a roller is fun and effective.

5. Move the muscle.

When you add motion to your Level 2 roller treatments, the treatment range for the unlocked muscles is instantly expanded. When you add active movement to the treatment, the muscles, tendons, and fascia are reset throughout a larger range of motion.

ROLLER PRE- AND POST-TESTS

If you're curious about the impact of a good roller treatment, try the following steps both before and after your roller exercises:

1. **Prior to rolling, walk across the room keeping your heels off the ground. Next, walk back to your starting spot keeping the front of your feet and toes up off the ground.**

2. **Perform three moderately deep two-legged body squats like you're sitting down in an imaginary low chair.**

3. **After your rolling treatment, compare changes in pain, tightness, and strength related to your knees, calves, and ankles asking yourself these questions:**

   - Are my lower leg muscles looser?
   - Do I feel less pressure on the front of your knees?
   - Has my ankle range of motion increased?
   - Do my lower legs feel stronger?

Unlocking the Calf — Back of Shin

"Calf" is a singular term, but a "calf muscle" is actually made up of two muscles. Those two muscles are the gastrocnemius muscle, the larger, more superficial muscle, and the soleus muscle, the deeper and shorter muscle, which is much closer to the two bones of the shin (see Figure 17-3).

The two calf muscles merge together to form the important Achilles tendon. When the two calf muscles contract, they pull the heel bone upward to push the foot off the ground. Meanwhile, they function quite differently, depending on the position of the knee.

The strong muscular gastrocnemius, or "gastroc," starts above the knee from two separate attachments on the back of the lower femur or thigh bone. The more slender and shorter soleus muscle starts well below the knee, attaching to the backside of the tibia and fibula, the two bones of the shin.

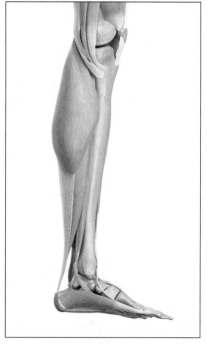

SciePro/Shutterstock

FIGURE 17-3:
The calf muscle includes the more superficial gastrocnemius and the deeper soleus muscles.

Because the gastroc originates *above* the knee, it is stronger when the knee is in full extension. The gastroc is also stretched more when the knee is in full extension. Conversely, because the soleus originates *below* the knee, the muscle is more isolated when the knee is bent or flexed.

Getting ready

As always, perform all roller treatments on a firmly padded surface with plenty of space to move around safely.

PT NOTE

Start by lying on your back, either resting back on your elbows or fully reclined. Bend the knee you will *not* be treating to approximately 90 degrees, with the foot flat and stable on the ground. On the calf you are treating, place the roller on the top ridge of the calf belly, just below the bend on the backside of the knee. Keep the elevated foot in a neutral position, in approximately 30 degrees of plantar (downward) flexion.

As you prepare to unlock or relax tight muscles, now is a good time to start your slow and deep breathing pattern.

TIP

Before you start any rolling treatment or exercise, it helps to quiet your body and mind. Close your eyes. Visualize your body resting in a relaxed and pain-free place. Perform three slow, deep breaths to prepare your body to heal.

The exercise

Here's how you can relax your calf muscles by unlocking their trigger points (see Figure 17-4).

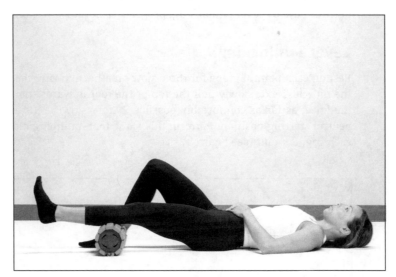

FIGURE 17-4:
Calf treatment with a roller.

Photography by Haim Ariav and Klara Cu

1. **Start by slowly moving the roller down the back of the calf muscle, by shifting your hips backwards.**

   Your objective is to find and crush painful trigger points, or "painful grapes," located throughout your calf muscles. Because the calf muscle is a wide muscle, you may have to guide the roller towards the inside or outside edge of the muscle belly.

TIP

   You can do this by simply pointing your toes to the left or the right. A fun way to do this is to visualize the face of a clock positioned below your foot. As you move the roller down the belly of your calf muscles, simply swing your toes anywhere between 10:00 and 2:00 on that imaginary clock face.

2. **Continue with loud breathing, slow rolling, and grape crushing down the back of the shin until you reach the finish line: approximately two inches above your Achilles tendon.**

Never roll on your Achilles tendon!

Level 1 unlocking

Rest on each trigger point for three slow breaths, allowing the roller to melt into the muscle like a hot knife through butter. Then resume the downward roll, seeking more trigger points.

If your calf muscles are both looser and pain-free with walking after a minimum of three days of Level 1 unlocking, progress to Level 2 unlocking.

Level 2 unlocking

Rest on each painful grape for three slow breaths, allowing the roller to melt into the muscle. Next, slowly pull the top of the foot upwards (dorsiflexion) towards the knee, as far as comfortably possible, before slowly returning the foot to its neutral starting position. Perform this slow, foot-pumping motion two times on each trigger point (see Figure 17-5).

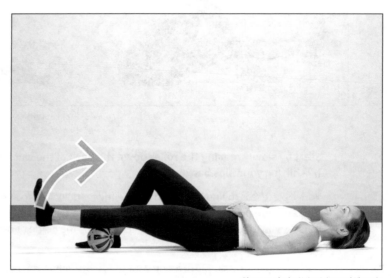

FIGURE 17-5: Level 2 calf treatment involves slowly pulling the foot upward two times on each trigger point.

Photography by Haim Ariav and Klara Cu

You'll quickly notice how much the muscle-unlocking intensity increases when Level 2 foot motion is added. Next, resume your seek-and-destroy mission down the calf, looking for the next painful grape.

Do's and don'ts

Keeping your calves happy is important for anyone who is active, stands for long parts of the day, and/or has a history of foot pain. For example, rolling too aggressively on a tight calf will make your pain worse and your calf muscles tighter. Here are the do's and don'ts for relaxing your calves without triggering a major lockdown of your fickle calf muscles.

>> Do breathe slow, deep, and loud.

>> Do move the roller in one direction: downward towards the ankle.

>> Do try other roller options, like vibrating rollers and roller balls, to determine the best ways to unlock your calf muscles (see Figure 17-6).

>> Do cross the other leg over the shin you are treating if additional weight is desired on the calf muscle during a treatment.

>> Don't roll your calf muscles too aggressively to avoid making your calf tighter.

>> Don't roll on an acutely strained calf muscle.

>> Don't roll on any area that produces numbness, tingling, shooting pain, or weakness.

>> Don't ignore deep calf pain that worsens with rest — it might be a blood clot!

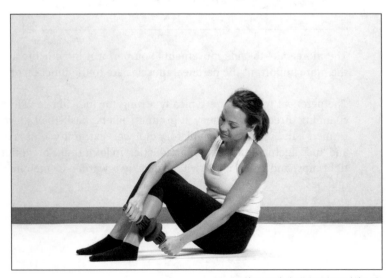

FIGURE 17-6:
Another option to work with rollers to relax lower leg muscles.

Photography by Haim Ariav and Klara Cu

Unlocking the Peroneals — Outside Corner of Lower Shin

For the sake of simplicity, I will focus on the two main peroneal muscles: the peroneus longus and the peroneus brevis. I will ignore the much less important weakling of the proud peroneal family, the peroneus tertius. The peroneal muscles are thin and lean, running down the back outside corners of the fibular bone. When the peroneals contract, they swing the foot outward to stabilize the outside of the ankle and foot. They serve an important function to control motion involving the outside of the ankle and foot (see Figure 17-7).

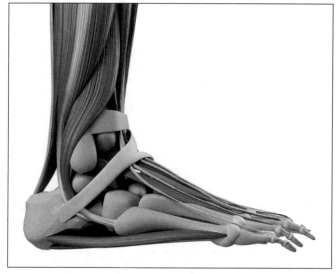

FIGURE 17-7: Getting to know your hidden peroneal muscles.

SciePro/Shutterstock

The more side-to-side movements you perform in your life and in your sports, the more important the peroneal muscles are to the function of your entire leg.

The peroneal muscles are typically strong for individuals who spend more time changing directions on uneven ground (hikers, basketball players, and off-road runners). Individuals with a history of lower-extremity joint laxity (ankle sprains and knee ligament injuries) or a reduction in joint range of motion (knee arthritis, tight hips, and stiff ankles) will be quickly rewarded by mobilizing their peroneal muscles.

Getting ready

As always, perform all roller treatments on a firmly padded surface with plenty of safe space to move around.

For the sake of understanding the directions of this treatment, let's talk about treating the *left* lower leg. Start by lying on your back, resting on your elbows. Bend your right knee to approximately 90 degrees, with your right foot flat on the ground. Place the roller just below the bottom outside ridge of your *left* calf belly. This should be approximately one-third of the way up the outer lower shin from the heel bone. Keep the ankle stable at an angle of approximately 90 degrees between the foot and the shin. Here comes the key to the proper starting position (again utilizing your imaginary clock): Rotate your entire left leg to the left so your middle toe is pointing to approximately 10:00 on your foot clock.

TIP

As you gain more experience with this very effective treatment technique, your starting leg angle may change. Based on your peroneal muscle tightness, calf size, and healing speed, you may find yourself rotating to, say, 9:30 or 10:45 to isolate certain chronic trigger points.

As you prepare to unlock or relax tight muscles, now is a good time to start your slow and deep breathing pattern.

TIP

Before you start any rolling treatment or exercise, it helps to quiet your body and mind. Close your eyes. Visualize your body resting in a relaxed and pain-free place. Perform three slow, deep breaths to prepare your body to heal.

The exercise

Here's how you can relax your peroneal muscles with a self-myofacial unlocking of their trigger points. The technique will sound a bit tricky at first. However, once you start finding the trigger points, adhesions, and restrictions, you will certainly know it, I promise.

1. **Start by slowly moving the roller down the back outside corner of your shin by shifting your hips backwards.**

   Your objective is to find and crush painful trigger points located along the back outside corner of the fibular bone, from just below the calf muscle belly down to the bottom of the ankle bone. You can do this by simply rotating the leg outward while using, as you did with the earlier calf treatment, your imaginary clock positioned below your foot (see Figure 17-8).

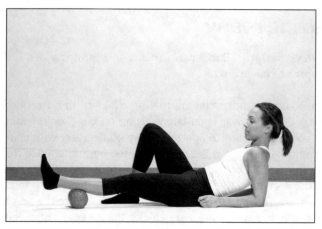

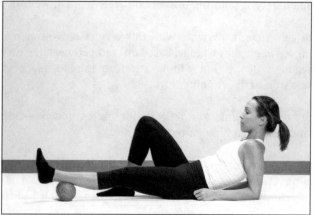

FIGURE 17-8:
Rolling the
peroneal
muscles:
start, middle,
and finishing
positions.

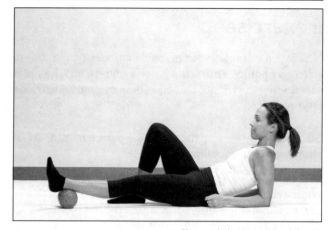

Photography by Haim Ariav and Klara Cu

In this example, the left leg is rotated outward or to the left. Remember to keep the ankle stable, at an angle of approximately 90 degrees between the foot and the shin.

2. **Keep rotating your entire left leg on your foot clock, pointing your middle toe between 9:30 and 11:00.**

This will help you find trigger points and adhesions as you roll down the peroneal muscles and tendons.

3. **Continue with loud breathing, slow rolling, and grape crushing down the back outside ridge of your fibular bone until you reach the finish line: the back bottom of your ankle bone.**

Level 1 unlocking

Rest on each trigger point for three slow breaths, allowing the roller to melt into the peroneal muscles like a hot knife through butter. Then resume the downward roll, seeking more trigger points. Keep rotating your entire leg in and out to expose more trigger points and adhesions.

If your peroneals and calf muscles are both looser and pain-free with walking after a minimum of three days of Level 1 unlocking, progress to Level 2 unlocking.

Level 2 unlocking

Rest on each painful grape for three slow breaths, allowing the roller to melt into the peroneal muscles. Next, while keeping your hip and knee stable and your ankle joint at a 90-degree angle, slowly swing *only your foot* side to side, approximately three to four inches in each direction. Perform this slow foot-swinging motion two times in each direction on each trigger point (see Figure 17-9).

You'll quickly notice how much the muscle-unlocking intensity increases when Level 2 foot motion is added. Next, resume your seek-and-destroy mission down the back outside ridge of the shin bone, looking for the next painful grape.

Do's and don'ts

Rolling your peroneal muscles and tendons can be uncomfortable. The following do's and don'ts will help you roll the outside of your lower shin properly while making it more comfortable.

>> Do breathe slow, deep, and loud.

>> Do move the roller in one direction: downward towards the outside of the ankle.

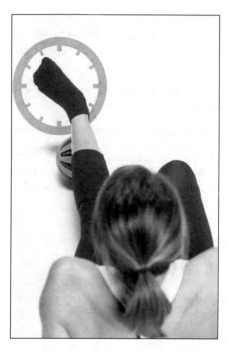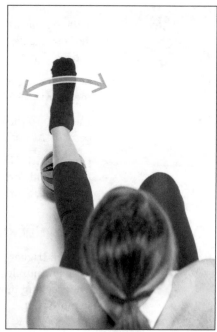

FIGURE 17-9: Level 2 peroneal treatments involve slowly swinging the foot inward and outward two times on each trigger point.

Photography by Haim Ariav and Klara Cu

>> Do play around with different shin and foot positions to adjust the amount of pressure and stretch applied to the muscles, tendons, and fascia.

>> Do try other roller options, like vibrating rollers and roller balls, to determine the best options to unlock your peroneal muscles. Warning: Tread slowly with smaller and harder rollers because these muscles and tendons can be painful to treat.

>> Do cross the other leg over the shin you're treating if additional weight is desired on peroneal muscles during a treatment.

>> Do try easy glides or sheering moves of the lower leg on the roller where restrictions are consistent to reduce fascial tissue tension.

>> Don't roll your peroneal muscles too aggressively.

>> Don't roll on a swollen lower shin.

>> Don't roll on any area that produces numbness, tingling, shooting pain, or weakness.

Unlocking the Ankle Dorsiflexors — Front of Shin

The main muscle on the front of the shin is called the anterior tibialis. Its main function is to pull the foot upwards towards the sky. This motion is referred to as *dorsiflexion*. There are two other small muscles that go to the toes, which help with this motion to a small degree. While the anterior tibialis is the big dog in this fight, all three muscles in the front of the shin will be treated with this technique. For the sake of simplicity, I will refer to these muscles simply as the dorsiflexors (see Figure 17-10).

Well, you might say, "The job of pulling my foot upward is not really important for me because I am neither a soccer player nor a punter on a football team."

Touché.

But let me give you two reasons why your ankle dorsiflexors are worth fighting for:

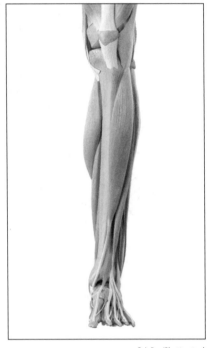

SciePro/Shutterstock

FIGURE 17-10:
The pride and glory of the front of the shin.

>> **They counterbalance your calf and Achilles tendon.** With a strong Achilles tendon formed by two strong calf muscles, it's hard to keep them flexible. A simple solution is to have strong, inflexible muscles on the opposite side of the joint, counterbalancing the strong gastroc, soleus, and Achilles tendon. In this case, the counterbalancing muscle is the anterior tibialis.

>> **They help you to maintain valuable ankle-range motion.** If your ankle dorsiflexors are weak and tight, they restrict your ankle joint motion. With that being said, a mobile ankle joint requires mobile muscles on both the front and back of the joint.

TIP

Before you start any rolling treatment or exercise, it helps to quiet your body and mind. Close your eyes. Visualize your body resting in a relaxed and pain-free place. Perform three slow, deep breaths to prepare your body to heal.

Getting ready

As always, perform all roller treatments on a firmly padded surface with plenty of safe space to move around.

For the sake of understanding the directions of this treatment, let's talk about treating the *left* lower leg.

Start by getting on your hands and knees. Place the roller just below your left knee on the front outside ridge of your upper shin. To do this, bend your left knee and tuck your left foot under your pelvis. The starting position for the roller is the upper anterior tibialis muscle belly. Keep your ankle stable at a 90-degree angle.

As you prepare to unlock or relax tight muscles, now is a good time to start your slow and deep breathing pattern.

OUCH

This position can be somewhat uncomfortable for someone with a stiff knee or tight lower back. Alter your position as needed by lying face-down with a straighter knee or using a chair to improve your balance.

The exercise

Here's how you can relax your ankle dorsiflexor muscles by unlocking their trigger points.

1. **Start by slowly moving the roller down the front of the shin by gliding your knee forward over the roller.**

   Your objective is to find and crush painful trigger points in the muscle bellies on the front of the shin (see Figure 17-11).

TIP

This treatment isn't the fuzzy and loving treatment you'll do to relax. It hurts, so start this technique slow and on a soft roller. After a long day on your feet, this treatment will help your shins and feet to recover faster before you hit the dance floor in the evening.

2. **Continue with loud breathing, slow rolling, and grape crushing down the front of the shin until you reach the finish line: your ankle joint.**

Level 1 unlocking

Rest on each trigger point for three slow breaths, allowing the roller to slowly melt into the shin muscles like a hot knife through butter. Then, resume the downward roll, seeking more trigger points.

If your ankle dorsiflexors are both looser and pain-free with walking after a minimum of three days of Level 1 unlocking, progress to Level 2 unlocking.

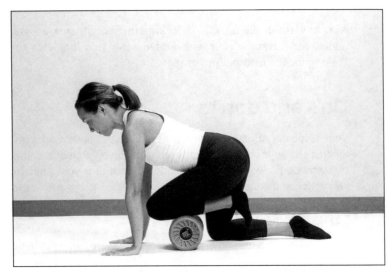

Photography by Haim Ariav and Klara Cu

FIGURE 17-11:
Rolling
the ankle
dorsiflexor
muscles.

Level 2 unlocking

Rest on each painful grape for three slow breaths, allowing the roller to melt into your dorsiflexor muscles. Next, slowly point your foot and toes downward as far as comfortably possible before slowly returning the foot to its dorsiflexed starting position. Perform this slow foot "pushing on the gas pedal" pumping motion two times on each trigger point (see Figure 17-12).

FIGURE 17-12:
Level 2
dorsiflexion
treatments
involve starting
with the
ankle at
90 degrees,
then pointing
the foot down
two times then
upwards on
each trigger
point.

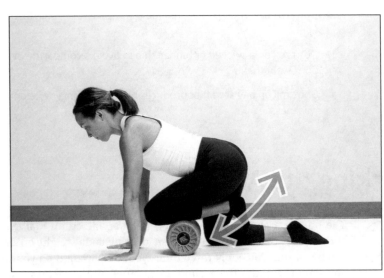

Photography by Haim Ariav and Klara Cu

Note how much the muscle-unlocking intensity increased when foot motion was added. Next, resume your seek-and-destroy mission down the front of the shin, looking for the next painful grape.

Do's and don'ts

Your ankle dorsiflexors on the front of the shin have a difficult task as they battle against the super strong calf muscles on the outside of the shin. This short list of do's and don'ts will keep "all hands on deck" for your ankle dorsiflexors to keep you active and pain-free.

>> Do breathe slow, deep, and loud.

>> Do move the roller in one direction: downward towards the front of the shin.

>> Do adjust different hip, knee, and shin positions to gain a comfortable position for your body. Don't forget my first rolling rule from Chapter 8: Align the spine.

>> Do try other roller options, like vibrating rollers, handheld massagers, and roller balls, to determine the best options to unlock your dorsiflexor muscles.

>> Do cross the other leg over your treating shin if additional weight is desired on the back of the peroneal muscles during a treatment.

>> Do try easy glides or sheering moves of the lower leg on the roller where restrictions are consistent to reduce fascial tissue tension.

>> Don't roll the front of your shin too aggressively. The shin fascia is naturally tight.

>> Don't roll on a swollen or tender shin to avoid a compartment syndrome. You don't want that!

>> Don't roll on any area that produces numbness, tingling, shooting pain, or weakness.

Unlocking the Arch

PT NOTE

The human arch (see Figure 17-13) is an architectural marvel! It supports your entire body, often with 100 percent of your body weight on only one arch. And when you run, you apply three times your body weight on your feet and arches as you slam them into the ground. I examined and treated thousands of huge professional football players during my 26-year NFL career. The largest NFL player I rehabbed weighed a whopping 404 pounds! Just think about the forces placed on his arches as he collided into other massive 330-plus-pound players on each and every play!

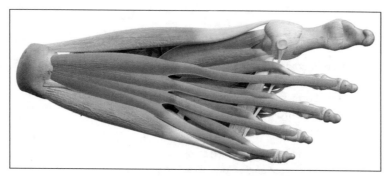

FIGURE 17-13:
The engineering marvel known as the human arch.

Each foot has 26 bones, countless ligaments holding those bones in the perfect position to withstand those high forces, and dozens of muscles supporting those loaded bones and ligaments. When you look at your relatively small feet that way, you can see why the muscles of the arch are so often tired and sore.

TIP

If you learn the simple roller ball tricks I'm about to show you for your arches, the roller ball will quickly raise to the status of Most Valuable Tool according to your feet. After a hard day of work or a workout, besides a bowl of Moose Tracks ice cream, nothing beats a foot massage with a roller ball!

Getting ready

Place a sturdy, supportive chair on a firm but non-slippery surface. Use a roller ball. If this is not available, use a lacrosse or golf ball inside a sock for extra padding. Lastly, have a three-plus-foot-long non-stretch nylon cord or band available for your Level 2 treatments.

Start by sitting comfortably in the sturdy chair on the non-slippery floor, demonstrating tall posture with your spine away from the back of the chair. With your knee bent to approximately 90 degrees, place the roller ball under the back part of your arch, just in front of your heel bone.

Cross your other leg across your bent knee so your upper shin is somewhat parallel to the floor. Place both palms on the upper horizontal shin to apply additional weight to the roller ball if needed.

Before you start any rolling treatment or exercise, it helps to quiet your body and mind. Close your eyes. Visualize your body resting in a relaxed and pain-free place. Perform three slow, deep breaths to prepare your body to heal.

The exercise

Here's how you can relax your arch muscles by unlocking their trigger points.

1. **Start by slowly moving the roller forward into your arch by gliding your heel backwards.**

   Try to keep your ankle close to a 90-degree angle. Your objective is to find and crush painful trigger points in your arch. This is easy to do, with most arches being over-worked and under-loved (see Figure 17-14).

2. **Continue with loud breathing, slow rolling in a small overlapping circular pattern and grape crushing in a forward direction until you reach the finish line: the bony underside of your toe joints.**

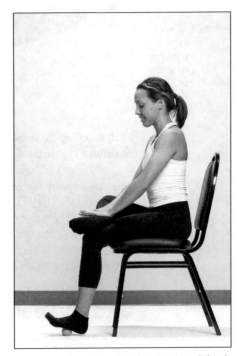

Photography by Haim Ariav and Klara Cu

FIGURE 17-14:
Rolling the arch with your Most Valuable Tool.

Depending on how wide your foot and roller ball are, some side-to-side shifting of the ball will help you roll your entire arch.

If extra pressure is desired, you're in a perfect position to use your hands to push downward to increase the force on the roller ball.

Level 1 unlocking

Rest on each trigger point for three slow breaths, allowing the roller ball to melt into the muscle like a hot knife through butter. Then resume the forward roll, seeking more trigger points.

If your arch muscles are both looser and pain-free with walking after a minimum of three days of Level 1 unlocking, progress to Level 2 unlocking.

Level 2 unlocking

Rest on each painful grape for three slow breaths, allowing the roller ball to melt into the muscles of the arch. Next, with the use of the non-stretch nylon cord or strap, use your arms to slowly pull the *toes* (not the foot) upward (extension) towards the knee, while keeping your ankle at a 90-degree angle. While pulling with the strap, engage the toes to assist with the lifting motion. Lift the toes as far as comfortably possible before allowing them to slowly return to their starting position. Perform this slow, active-assistive extension motion two times on each trigger point (see Figure 17-15).

Note the increased intensity of the arch muscles unlocking when toe stretching is added. Next, resume your seek-and-destroy mission down the arch, looking for the next trigger point or adhesion.

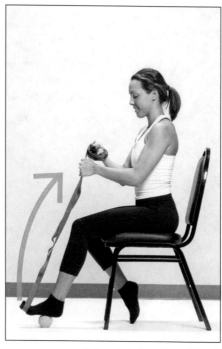

Photography by Haim Ariav and Klara Cu

FIGURE 17-15:
Level 2 arch treatments involve a non-stretch cord to assist the stretching of the toe flexor tendons.

Do's and don'ts

I want to share a few tips for a heavenly arch massage before a big workout or after a tough day of work:

- » Do breathe slow, deep, and loud.

- » Do move the roller in one direction: forward towards the toes.

- » Do adjust different knee and foot positions to expose additional trigger points and adhesions.

- » Do try other roller options, like vibrating rollers, handheld massagers, and roller balls, to determine the best ways to unlock your dorsiflexor muscles.

- » Do cross the other leg over your treating shin if additional weight is desired on the arch muscles during a treatment.

» Do try easy glides or sheering moves of the arch on the roller where restrictions are consistent to reduce fascial tissue tension.

» Don't roll your heel bone, the ball of your foot under your big toe, or any bony landmarks on the underside of your foot.

» Don't be too aggressive in starting the position in the back of the arch if you have a history of plantar fasciitis. This is a great treatment for that painful injury, but start slowly to learn how your arch responds to this technique.

» Don't roll on any area that produces numbness, tingling, shooting pain, or weakness.

IN THIS CHAPTER

» Appreciating the complexity and value of the lumbar spine, pelvis, and hip regions

» Treating your lumbar spine safely and effectively

» Seeing and feeling how the hip flexors impact your entire body

» Understanding why your hip external rotators are so tight and learning how to loosen them

» Treating your glute pain quickly and effectively

Chapter **18**

Unlocking Your Lower Back and Hips

Lower back pain is no joke. In fact, way too many people suffer from pain in their lumbar spine. When we combine hip pain with lower back pain, it's safe to say, this chapter may help eliminate more pain than any other chapter in this book. I truly hope so, because I've watched crippling lower back pain ruin way too many lives.

PT NOTE

There are a lot of important moving parts in the lower back, pelvis, and hip joint. Because of the complexity involving bones, joints, muscles, tendons, ligaments, and fascia, even small compensations in the lower back, pelvis, and hip result in large body compensations elsewhere.

I think it's extremely important to keep the medical information and physical therapy techniques for these body parts simple. My focus in this chapter is to help you move better with less pain, not to make you an anatomy expert. When my anatomy and kinesiology geek tendencies start to surface, I remind myself to "keep it simple, Mike."

REMEMBER

Play around with the exercises in this chapter and see what works best for you. Perform the pre-test of marching and squatting to assess where you're feeling tightness, pain, or restrictions. Treat those areas with the techniques in this chapter, starting slowly. Then, reassess your movement with the same post-test to compare how you move after the treatments. Determine what helped and what hurt. Document your new plan and get busy moving better every day.

Ryan Rolling Rules for Your Hips and Lower Back

REMEMBER

In Chapter 8 we went in great details regarding the value of applying my five Ryan Rolling Rules for all our roller treatments. The five rules are simple to apply and make your roller treatments safer and much more effective. The safety factor becomes extremely important when we apply the roller to parts of your body involving your spine. For example, if you're rolling your lumbar spine or hip and the 24 vertebral bones in your spine are poorly aligned, your spine pain could quickly get worse not better!

I suggest you flip back to Chapter 8 for a quick review before you start these lower back and hip roller treatments. Following is an abbreviated version of those five rules:

1. Align the spine.

Proper posture on the roller is a must. Even when you're rolling the bottom of the spine, maintaining a straight and stable spine from your pelvis to your skull will protect the entire spine.

2. Breathe.

If you hold your breath while rolling, which is a natural response when in pain, the outcome of your roller treatments will suffer. Stated bluntly, if you're a bad breather, you'll be a bad roller. Being a good breather is easy: Inhale and exhale slowly, deeply, and loudly.

3. Slow roll. Rolling at a slow speed gives your body more time for positive changes to occur. This is especially true when rolling larger, stronger muscles closer to the spine.

ROLLER PRE- AND POST-TEST

Use this test to help you immediately feel the benefits of rolling while evaluating your rolling techniques:

1. **Prior to rolling, march across the room with high-knee steps like you're marching across a field of waist-high grass.**

2. **Perform three moderately deep two-legged body squats like you're sitting down in an imaginary low chair.**

3. **After your rolling treatment, compare changes in pain, tightness, and strength related to your low back, pelvis, and hips by asking yourself these questions:**

- Are my lower back and hip muscles looser?

- Do I feel less pressure across my lower back?

- Does it feel like my hips are looser?

- Do I now have more control of my pelvis when I move?

4. **Seek and destroy.**

   Imagine yourself driving a military mine sweeper over your lower back and hips. Your mission: Seeking painful trigger points and adhesions throughout your backside landscape and destroying them! We all know how limiting lower back and hip trigger points and adhesions can be.

5. **Move the muscle.**

   During all our Level 2 roller treatments, we add active movements to accelerate the unlocking of tight muscles and to expand your joint range of motion. When your pain-free movement patterns increase, regardless of how expansive those motions are, your muscles, tendons and fascia stop protecting your movements.

An Inside Look at the Lower Back and Hips

If you have difficulty determining if your pain or tightness is coming from your lower back or your hip, you're not alone. Separating the lumbar spine from the pelvis from the hip joint is no easy task, even for medical experts. Yet all three of these major body structures — the spine, pelvis, and hip — are no more than eight inches apart (see Figure 18-1).

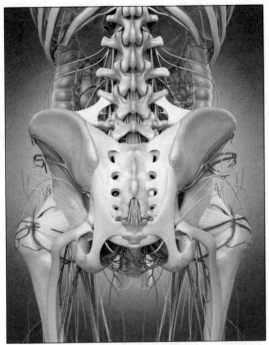

FIGURE 18-1:
Anatomy of the lower back and hip region.

SciePro/Shutterstock

I'll provide individualized introductions for each of the four body parts — the lower back, hip flexors, hip external rotators, and glutes — in this chapter. You will learn about and understand each of the four parts separately. But the greatest gift of this chapter will be you understanding how these four important body parts work together. This synergy, where "the whole is greater than the sum of its parts," can help you improve how your lower back and hips move and function.

TIP

The lower back directly impacts the hip joint, and the hip joint directly impacts the lower back. Therefore, using a quick pre-test and post-test for your lower back and hip joint treatments is the smart thing to do. Comparing how well you walk and squat before and after a lower-back roller treatment will help you determine if the majority of your pain is truly coming from your lumbar spine. Conversely, performing those same pre-tests and post-tests with simple walking and squatting assessments before and after your hip roller treatments will help you confirm whether your hip is the epicenter of your pain.

"MYSTERIOUS" HIP PAIN

For most people, when it comes to hip pain, the first word that comes to mind is "mysterious." I say this because most people with hip pain have few clues to the source of their pain. The typical pattern of their hip pain goes like this:

- Their hip just gets tight for no specific reason.

- They are forced to limit their activity level and hope the pain will go away.

- Weeks or months later, they're still limping.

- Reluctantly, they go to their doctor for an exam and X-ray.

- "You have some arthritis but your hip isn't fractured" becomes their lame diagnosis.

- Everyone keeps telling them, "You have a bad hip."

- They're still limping, still in pain, and still in the dark.

- Sadly, the "mystery" lives on.

I became angry writing this list. I've evaluated and treated way too many patients, friends, and family who were forced down that same painful rabbit hole. Many of them failed to ever get clear direction regarding the source of their pain. They were left to journey down this painful road, confused and alone. I don't rest the blame for their situations solely on their healthcare providers. The patient, too, is responsible to seek prompt answers and to play an *active*, not passive, role seeking both the source of the pain *and* a recovery specialists. Ideally, this is a team process involving the patient, medical specialists, family, and caring friends.

I really enjoy treating patients with lumbar spine and hip issues because the complexity of their functional anatomy is a great challenge for me. And when we, not "I", unravel the mystery of their pain and devise an effective recovery plan for these patients, their life can change instantly. It's amazing to watch!

Unlocking the Lower Back — Back Extensors

Filled with rock-hard bones, strong muscles, stabilizing ligaments, tight fascia, and important nerves, your lower back is a very busy part of your body. Sticking to my game plan to "keep it simple," let's focus on treating the many strong muscles and tight fascia of the lumbar spine region, as shown in Figure 18-2.

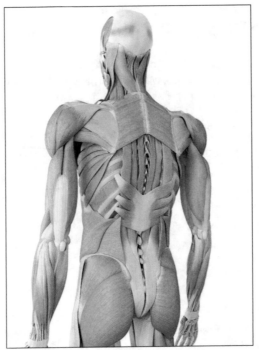

FIGURE 18-2:
Anatomy of the
lower back.

SciePro/Shutterstock

Before you start any roller treatments in this area, I want to remind you to protect your nerves. What I mean by this is to focus on treating the muscles and fascia without injuring the many nerves throughout this area. To do this, avoid creating what we call "nerve pain." If you're rolling on a painful spot that sends shooting pain down the leg, similar to the "funny bone" symptoms in your elbow, remove the roller pressure immediately. The symptoms from roller nerve pressure can include numbness, shooting pain, pins and needles, and muscle weakness below the point of contact.

The roller treatments involving the lower back use the roller to find areas of tightness and adhesions to reduce their restrictions. Many small, yet strong, muscles are located along the backside of the lumbar spine and pelvis. Taking your time to scan this area to find trigger points will be your game plan.

OUCH

As I note in the "Do's and Don'ts" section and in Chapter 5, you should always protect your spine. Avoid simply lying over the roller with it placed across the lumbar spine. This posture puts your lower back into an extreme extended posture that is dangerous for the lumbar spine and sacroiliac joints.

Getting ready

As always, perform all roller treatments on a firmly padded surface with plenty of safe space to move around.

PT NOTE

Start by lying on your back, on your solid, padded rolling surface. Place the roller ball or half-roller under your lower back just above the top of your glutes, as shown in Figure 18-3. Because you will often be rolling and shifting while treating your lower back, having extra pillows, pads, or towels will help keep your hands and elbows more comfortable.

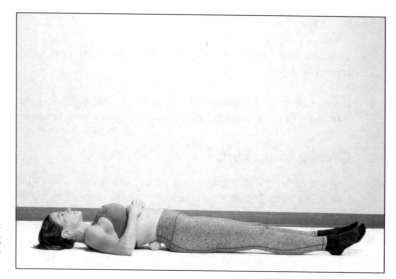

FIGURE 18-3:
Positioning for rolling the lower back.

Photography by Haim Ariav & Klara Cu

TIP

Before you start any rolling treatment or exercise, it helps to quiet your body and mind. Close your eyes. Visualize your body resting in a relaxed and pain-free place. Perform three slow, deep breaths to prepare your body to heal.

The exercise

Here's how you can relax your lower back muscles by unlocking their trigger points.

Level 1 unlocking

Rest on each trigger point for three slow breaths, allowing the roller ball or half roller to melt into the muscle like a hot knife through butter. Then resume the upward and sideward rolls, seeking more trigger points. Because you're treating a wider area with a narrow roller, continue to return to the top half of your pelvis bone to slightly alter the upward path of your roller ball like a broom.

TIP

To help your overlapping lower-back rolling technique, envision how you would sweep a wide, dusty hallway with a narrow broom:

1. **Anchor the broom.**

2. **Sweep.**

3. **Re-anchor the broom in a slightly different position.**

4. **Repeat.**

Continue with loud breathing and slow rolling from your beltline upward to your lower rib region.

If your lower back muscles are both looser and pain-free with walking after a minimum of three days of Level 1 unlocking, progress to Level 2 unlocking.

Level 2 unlocking

Rest on each "painful grape" for three slow breaths, allowing the roller ball or half roller to melt into the muscle. ("Painful grapes" is my whimsical name for these localized muscle restrictions.) Next, slowly add an abdominal crunch on top of the roller ball while exhaling for a count of three seconds, as shown in Figure 18-4. Slowly return your torso to its neutral starting position. Perform this slow abdominal crunch move two times on each trigger point.

You'll quickly notice how much the muscle-unlocking intensity increases when Level 2 core motion is added. Next, resume your seek-and-destroy mission throughout the lower back, looking for the next painful grape.

Do's and don'ts

Here are your do's and don'ts to roll your back extensor muscles effectively and safely. With many strong muscles along with plenty of sensitive nerves in your low back, these tips will help you know where to roll and where not to roll.

>> Do breathe slowly, deeply, and loudly.

>> Do move the roller slowly while keeping your spine well aligned.

>> Do try other roller options, like vibrating rollers, half rollers, and roller balls, to determine the best ways to unlock your lumbar spine muscles.

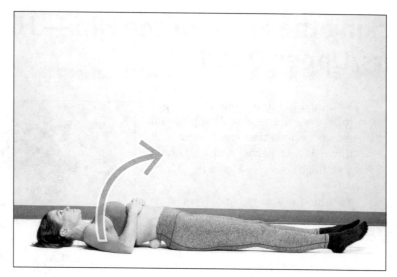

FIGURE 18-4:
Level 2
lower-back
treatments
involve adding
two crunches
on each trigger
point.

Photography by Haim Ariav and Klara Cu

>> Do use towels, pillows, or pads to support weight-bearing body parts and to protect your elbows.

>> Don't roll on your spine bones or pelvis bones.

>> Don't lie over the roller, placing your lower spine into extreme extension.

>> Don't roll on any area that produces numbness, tingling, shooting pain, or weakness.

PT NOTE

TREATING A PROFESSIONAL FOOTBALL PLAYER WITH LOW BACK PAIN CAUSED BY A HIDDEN HIP PROBLEM

Another reason why I love to treat patients with lower back and hip issues is because the "fixes" can be quick and long lasting. For example, you'd be amazed at how many patients I've "cured" with a $2.00 felt heel lift, simply because they had one leg longer than the other. One of my NFL professional football players came to me with severe, chronic lower-back pain that he'd suffered with since high school. He was an all-star Pro Bowl player and played in the NFL Super Bowl with his previous team. In other words, he was one of the best players in the league. During my physical therapy evaluation, I was shocked to find that one of his legs was over an inch longer than the other one. No one had ever discovered this during all his previous medical exams. I made him custom foot orthotics with a built-in heel lift. His lumbar spine pain disappeared in three days!

Unlocking the Front of the Hip — Hip Flexors/Upper Quad

Your three hip flexor muscles help you to be very active because these powerful muscles extend from your lower back through your pelvis, and anchor on your thigh bone (see Figure 18-5).

TIP

Your hip flexors are big players when it comes to the power associated with the front of your hips. Your hip flexors are comprised of three separate muscles: the powerful psoas major and iliacus along with the smaller psoas minor.

PT NOTE

I also include the "upper quad" with the hip flexors. To be specific, I'm including the rectus femoris muscle, which is one of the four (hence the name "quad") quadriceps muscles. The rectus femoris (or simply "rectus") is the only quad muscle that crosses the hip joint. The other three muscles of the quad anchor on the upper femur, or thigh bone, below the hip joint.

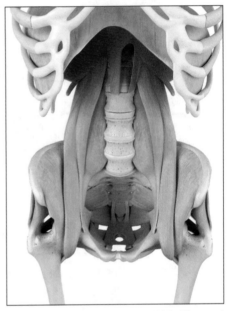

SciePro/Shutterstock

FIGURE 18-5:
Anatomy of the hip flexors.

REMEMBER

For clarity, when we say we're treating the hip flexor, we're focusing on the Big Three: psoas major, iliacus, and rectus femoris. These three strong muscles assist in lifting the thigh bone up towards the abdomen. With that being said, when the hip flexor becomes tight and inflexible, these strong muscles lock down the hip and restrict the hip's ability to extend or push off when walking, climbing stairs, and running.

Getting ready

As always, perform all roller treatments on a firmly padded surface with plenty of safe space to move around.

Lie face down towards the top half of your launch pad. Place a full roller, half roller, or roller ball just above your beltline on only one side of your navel, as shown in Figure 18-6. Rest comfortably on your chest or on both elbows in a plank-like position.

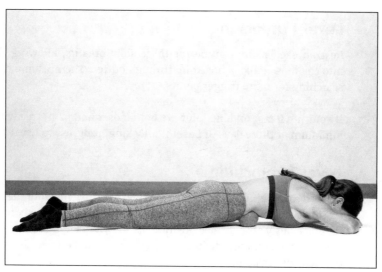

Photography by Haim Ariav and Klara Cu

If this starting position is uncomfortable for your knees or elbows, use pillows or towels to support your body weight.

REMEMBER

Before you start any rolling treatment or exercise, it helps to quiet your body and mind. Close your eyes. Visualize your body resting in a relaxed and pain-free place. Perform three slow, deep breaths to prepare your body to heal.

The exercise

Here's how you can relax your hip flexor muscles by unlocking their trigger points.

PT NOTE

1. Start by slowly rolling yourself upward, allowing the roller to glide downward over the hip joint.

2. By moving your elbows upward, slowly move the roller down towards the front of the thigh, searching for trigger points and areas of tightness.

3. With continuous deep breathing, find all the painful grapes between your lower abdomen and upper thigh and crush them.

4. Use the other leg and your elbows to rotate your pelvis and torso as one, to find adhesions and tightness across the entire front half of your hip joint.

5. Continue with loud breathing and slow rolling down the inner thigh until you reach the finish line: your mid-thigh.

Level 1 unlocking

Rest on each painful grape for three slow breaths, allowing the roller to melt into the muscle like a hot knife through butter. Then resume the downward roll, searching for more trigger points.

If your hip flexor and hip joint are both looser and pain-free with walking after a minimum of three days of Level 1 unlocking, progress to Level 2 unlocking.

Level 2 unlocking

Rest on each painful grape for three slow breaths, allowing the roller to melt into the muscle. Next, slowly lift the roller leg approximately six inches while maintaining a fairly straight-leg position, as shown in Figure 18-7. Slowly return to the starting position until the toes touch the ground. Perform this slow lift two times on each trigger point.

Note how much the muscle-unlocking intensity increases when hip extension is added. Next, resume your seek-and-destroy mission across the front of your hip, looking for the next painful grape.

Do's and don'ts

Here are some do's and don'ts for rolling your hips:

- >> Do breathe slow, deep, and loud.
- >> Do be creative while you roll; change the knee and hip angles to alter the length of your anterior hip muscles.
- >> Do move the roller slowly while keeping your spine well aligned.
- >> Do try other roller options, like vibrating rollers, half rollers, handheld massagers, and roller balls, to determine the best ways to unlock your hip flexors and upper quad.
- >> Do use towels, pillows, or pads to support weight-bearing body parts and to protect your elbows.
- >> Don't roll on painful abdominal areas, surgical sites, or your pelvis bone.
- >> Don't roll on any area that produces numbness, tingling, shooting pain, or weakness.

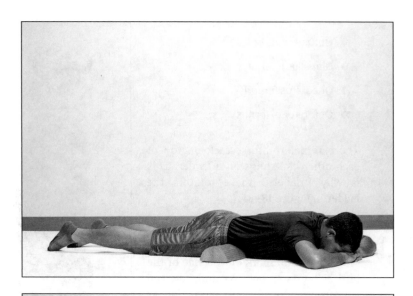

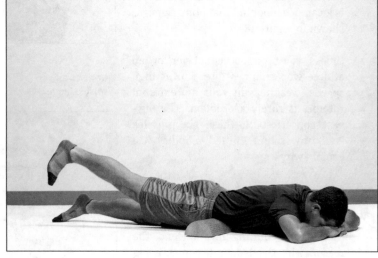

Photography by Haim Ariav and Klara Cu

FIGURE 18-7:
Level 2
hip flexor
treatments
involve adding
a slow leg lift
of six inches,
then returning
the toes to the
ground two
times on each
trigger point.

Unlocking the Side of the Hip — Hip External Rotators, aka "The Ladder"

Your hips have six external rotators that, you guessed it, rotate your thigh bone outward. They are:

>> Piriformis

>> Gemellus superior

>> Obturator internus

>> Gemellus inferior

>> Quadratus femoris

>> Obturator externus

The external rotators stack on top of each other like rungs on a ladder. This is why I labeled these rotators the ladder in Figure 18-8.

PT NOTE

This ladder is located beside your butt (or glute) muscles. Feel for the bony "hip bone" landmark on the side of the hip, below your beltline and between your front and back pockets. The ladder is located just behind that bony ridge, as shown in Figure 18-9.

Unless you're a soccer player or an athlete who changes direction at high speeds, weakness in your hip external rotators is rarely a problem. The biggest concern with these six muscles is tightness and limited mobility. I'll explain why.

PT NOTE

External rotators rotate the leg *outward*. When those same muscles become tight and restricted, they drastically limit the leg from rotating *inward*. Hence the reason why the ladder becomes a big source of pain and compensations for athletes young and old.

TIP

The next time you walk out of the shower, through a puddle, or across the pool deck, turn around and look at your wet footprints. Are both of your feet parallel and pointing in the exact same direction you are walking? Probably not. I bet your feet are slightly externally or laterally rotated.

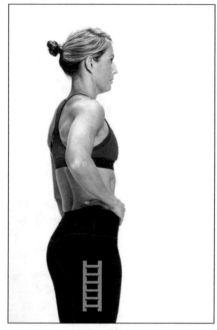

Photography by Haim Ariav and Klara Cu

FIGURE 18-8:
A trusted ladder.

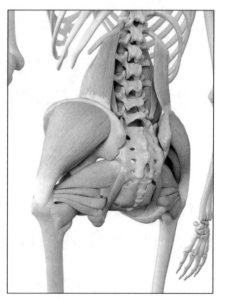

SciePro/Shutterstock

FIGURE 18-9:
A closer look at the "ladder": the hip external rotators.

Following are some common leg (and therefore hip) positions:

Position/Activity	Hip Position
Sitting at desk	Externally rotated
Sitting in car	Externally rotated
Standing	Externally rotated
Sleeping on back	Externally rotated
Sleeping on stomach	Externally rotated
Sleeping on side	Internally rotated
Walking	Slightly externally rotated
Biking	Slightly externally rotated
Running — distance	Slightly externally rotated
Running — sprinting	Internally rotated
Bull riding	Externally rotated

TIP

Pull out a pen and paper and calculate how many hours per day your hips are in an externally rotated position. Make a note to monitor your hips and legs throughout the day to see what position they're most comfortable in. You'll quickly come to agree with me: "Our hip external rotators are way too tight!"

PT NOTE

This is another reason why I love using half rollers and roller balls on this part of the body. I'll show you my tricks to unlock your ladder to gain pain-free internal hip rotation in less than five minutes.

One last point I want to share is why we need to keep our ladders unlocked and flexible. Take a guess at what part of our anatomy weaves right through (not over or under) the ladder.

OUCH

The sciatic nerve! If your ladder is tight, guess what it does to your sciatic nerve? A tight group of hip external rotators acts like a guillotine as it cinches down on the large sciatic nerve while it attempts to pass down the back-lateral thigh towards the lower leg.

How many people do you know who are walking around with pain down their leg or who have been given the generic diagnosis of "sciatica" but without a recovery plan? The truth is the source of their pain is often treatable pressure on their sciatic nerve. This is where the roller ball becomes very effective if used properly to unlock muscles applying unnecessary pressure on the sciatic nerve.

Getting ready

As always, perform all roller treatments on a firmly padded surface with plenty of safe space to move around.

Here are two key points I want to make before you start this treatment:

>> You should be clear on the location of your hip external rotators. You can review the details in the previous section and also Figure 18-9.

>> This treatment is best performed with either a half roller or a roller ball. A full-size roller is usually too large to properly isolate these deep, small muscles.

Start by lying on your back or reclined on your elbows, with one leg bent and that foot placed firmly on the ground. Place the half roller on the ladder, just behind your hip bone, with the half roller aligned parallel to your thigh bone, as shown in Figure 18-10.

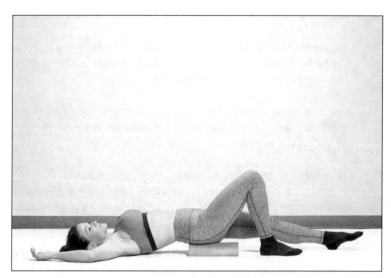

FIGURE 18-10: Starting position for treating hip external rotators.

Photography by Haim Ariav and Klara Cu

Before you start any rolling treatment or exercise, it helps to quiet your body and mind. Close your eyes. Visualize your body resting in a relaxed and pain-free place. Perform three slow, deep breaths to prepare your body to heal.

The exercise

Here's how you can relax your hip external rotator muscles by unlocking their trigger points.

1. **Start by slowly shifting more body weight onto the half roller through your hip external rotators.**

2. **Slowly straighten and bend your knee to move the pressure of the half roller up and down the ladder.**

   This is what I refer to as "walking up and down the ladder," as you fish for tender trigger points.

3. **Maintain loud, deep breathing as you walk up and down the ladder.**

Level 1 unlocking

Rest on each painful grape for three slow breaths, allowing the roller to melt into the hip rotator muscles like a hot knife through butter. Resume knee extension and flexion, seeking more trigger points and areas of tightness.

If your hip external rotator muscles are both looser and pain-free with walking after a minimum of three days of Level 1 unlocking, progress to Level 2 unlocking.

Level 2 unlocking

Rest on each painful grape for three slow breaths, allowing the half roller or roller ball to melt into the muscles. Next, slowly allow the bent knee to swing outward towards the floor. This is what I refer to as "opening the gate." Then, swing the leg upward ("closing the gate"), returning to the starting position, as shown in Figure 18-11. Perform "opening the gate/closing the gate" two times on each trigger point.

Note how much the muscle-unlocking intensity increases when the leg swinging motion is added.

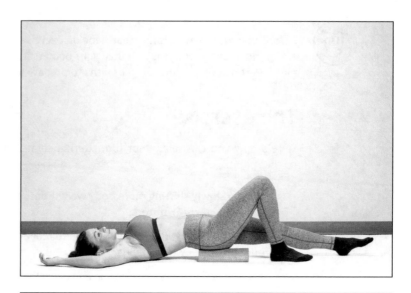

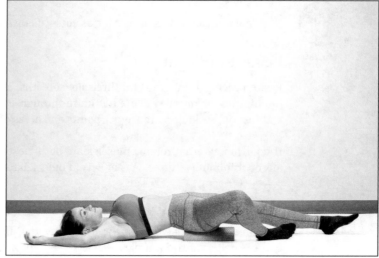

Photography by Haim Ariav and Klara Cu

FIGURE 18-11:
Level 2 hip external rotator treatment involves adding "opening the gate" and "closing the gate" with the treated leg two times on each trigger point.

Do's and don'ts

Treating your tight hip external rotators by "walking up and down the ladder" is a great way to quickly loosen up the back lower half of your hip joint. As you look back at Figure 18-1, you'll appreciate how busy that area is, including big, sensitive nerves. The following do's and don'ts will help you navigate the mind-field of the back of the hip joint, helping you put roller pressure exactly where you need it.

- >> Do breathe slow, deep, and loud.

- >> Do be creative while you roll; change knee and hip angles to alter the length of your hip external rotators.

- >> Do move the roller slowly while keeping your spine well aligned.

- >> Do use the wall to treat the ladder in a weight-bearing posture, as shown in Figure 18-12.

- >> Do try other roller options, like vibrating rollers, handheld massagers, and roller balls, to determine the best ways to unlock your hip rotators.

- >> Don't roll on bony hip or pelvis bones.

- >> Don't lie on hip external rotators and the sciatic nerve for more than one continuous minute.

- >> Don't roll on any area that produces numbness, tingling, shooting pain, or weakness.

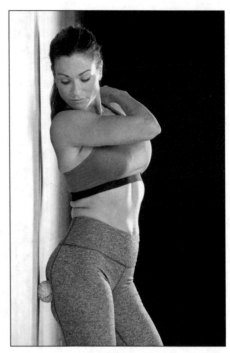

Photography by Haim Ariav and Klara Cu

FIGURE 18-12:
Using the wall is another option to "walk up and down the ladder" to relieve sciatic pain by unlocking hip external rotator muscles.

Unlocking the Back of the Hip — The Glutes, aka "The Roof"

The following three powerful hip extensors are collectively referred to as the glutes:

- >> Gluteus maximus — Daddy Bear

- >> Gluteus medius — Momma Bear

- >> Gluteus minimus — Baby Bear

The three glute muscles, shown in Figure 18-13, originate in the large concavity on the back half of the pelvis. The smaller gluteus minimus is the deepest, the gluteus medius is the middle glute, and the biggest glute, gluteus maximus, is the most superficial. The three glutes overlap each other as they travel down and outward, anchoring on the top of the thigh bone.

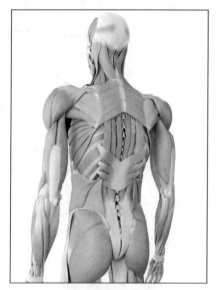

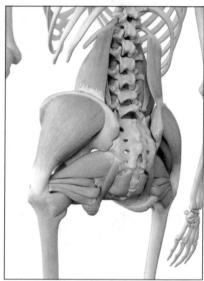

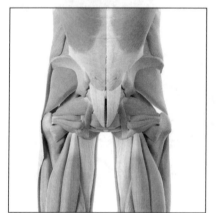

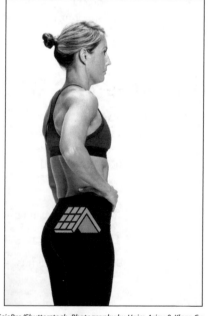

FIGURE 18-13: The anatomy of the "roof": the three glute muscles.

SciePro/Shutterstock, Photography by Haim Ariav & Klara Cu

Based on their layered positions and shape, I collectively refer to the glutes as "the roof." When strong and active, the glutes proudly protrude out over the back of the hip joint like the eve of a roof.

REMEMBER

The thick, strong glutes counteract the function of the mighty hip flexors on the opposite side of the pelvis: the hip flexors up front flex the hip, while the glutes on the backside extend the hip. These two pelvis superpowers strongly depend upon each other for a full hip range of motion.

The glutes do more than just extend the hip. They assist with stabilizing the pelvis over the leg when walking, running, and changing directions. They assist with hip rotation. They even support the function of the iliotibial band at the knee.

PT NOTE

But with broad function comes the potential for broad dysfunction. With the three glute muscles strategically nestled between the hips, the sacrum's sacroiliac joints, and the base of the entire spine, the glutes are certainly in a busy neighborhood. I often think of the glutes as being similar to the grassy middle median between two sides of Germany's Autobahn superhighway. There certainly is a lot going on all around the glutes.

OUCH

Because of their many roles and busy location, even small trigger points, adhesions, and restrictions involving the three glutes will be painful and immediately limiting for the lumbar spine, pelvis, and hip.

PT NOTE

I love treating the roof with a roller ball. As with the hip rotators, a full-size roller can be too large to apply deep pressure to all three glute muscles. You're welcome to start with a full-size roller or half roller if it helps you master the technique before progressing to the firmer and smaller roller ball.

The glutes are easy to treat with a roller ball for many reasons:

>> Glute muscles are easy to find.

>> The spine is well supported with this treatment.

>> Muscles have a hard, bony backstop.

>> Glutes are a hotbed for trigger points.

>> Only a small active motion is needed for Level 2 treatments.

>> Unlocking the three glutes produces immediate relief.

Getting ready

As always, perform all roller treatments on a firmly padded surface with plenty of safe space to move around.

Start by lying on your back or reclining on elbows with one leg bent and the foot of that leg placed firmly on the ground. Place the roller ball on the top half of the roof, which is the larger glute muscle belly just below your beltline, as shown in Figure 18-14.

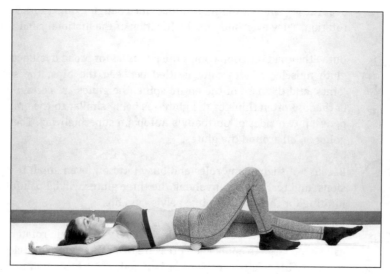

FIGURE 18-14: Starting position for glute muscle treatments.

REMEMBER

Before you start any rolling treatment or exercise, it helps to quiet your body and mind. Close your eyes. Visualize your body resting in a relaxed and pain-free place. Perform three slow, deep breaths to prepare your body to heal.

The exercise

Here's how you can relax your glute muscles by unlocking their trigger points.

1. **Start by slowly shifting more body weight onto the roller ball through your glute muscles.**

2. **Slowly shift your pelvis and spine in a circular pattern as you use the roller ball to scan through your glute muscle bellies.**

   This is what I refer to as "walking around the roof." It won't take long before you find a few painful trigger points that will make you groan and your palms start to sweat.

Alternate option: Form a "figure four," with your treated leg's ankle resting on the thigh of the other leg's bent knee, as shown in Figure 18-15. This position puts the hip joint in a flexed and externally rotated position, stretching the ladder. In this position, place the roller, the half roller, or, if you truly love pain, the roller ball under the roof. As I described earlier, start your circular scanning movement to seek and destroy trigger points and adhesions.

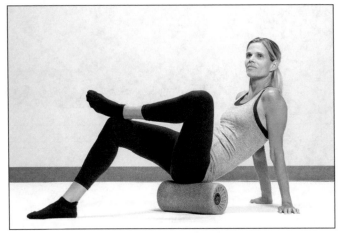

FIGURE 18-15:
Alternate
figure-four
position for
rolling the roof.

Photography by Haim Ariav and Klara Cu

REMEMBER

Maintain loud, deep breathing as you walk around the roof.

Level 1 unlocking

Rest on each painful trigger point for three slow breaths, allowing the roller ball to melt into the muscles like a hot knife through butter. Then resume the circular scanning movement, seeking more trigger points and areas of tightness. Try changing your knee and hip angles to make the roof larger or smaller, altering the length of the three glute muscles.

If your glute muscles are both looser and pain-free with walking after a minimum of three days of Level 1 unlocking, progress to Level 2 unlocking.

Level 2 unlocking

Rest on each painful grape for three slow breaths, allowing the roller ball to melt into the glute muscles. Next, slowly allow the bent knee to swing outward towards the floor, as shown in Figure 18-16. This is what I refer to as "opening the gate." Next, swing the leg upward ("closing the gate"), returning to the starting position. Perform opening and closing the gate two times on each trigger point.

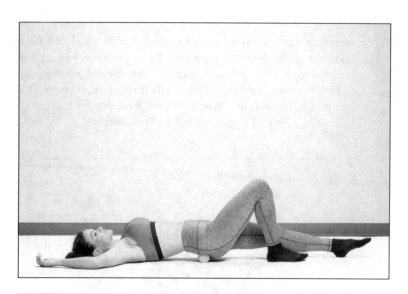

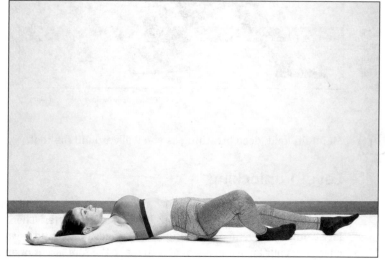

Photography by Haim Ariav and Klara Cu

FIGURE 18-16: Level 2 glute muscle treatments, "opening the gate" and "closing the gate."

Note how much the muscle-unlocking intensity increases when the leg swinging motion is added.

Do's and don'ts

"Walking around the roof" with a roller ball or roller is the perfect way to perform a self-myofascial unlocking of your three glute muscles. When you get really good at this treatment, don't act surprised when "that low back-hip kinda thing" just seems to disappear. Use the following tips to help you perform your magical pain disappearing act:

>> Do breathe slow, deep, and loud.

>> Do know where your three glute muscles are located, as represented by the "roof" in Figure 18-17a.

>> Do be creative while you roll; change knee and hip angles to alter the length of your glute muscles.

>> Do use the wall to treat the roof in a weight-bearing posture (see Figure 18-17b).

>> Do move the roller slowly while keeping your spine well aligned.

>> Do try other roller options, like vibrating rollers and half rollers, to determine the best ways to unlock your glutes.

>> Don't roll on bony hip or pelvis bones.

>> Don't lie on hip external rotators and the sciatic nerve for more than one continuous minute.

>> Don't roll on any area that produces numbness, tingling, shooting pain, or weakness.

FIGURE 18-17: Using the wall is another option to "walk around the roof" to eliminate lower back pain caused by glute-muscle trigger points.

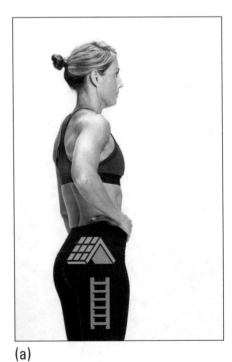

(a)

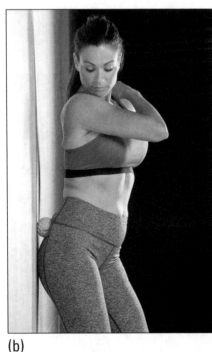

(b)

Photography by Haim Ariav and Klara Cu

Chapter **19**

Unlocking Your Chest, Upper Back, and Neck

The top half of your spine is the key to your body posture. A forward head, tight chest muscles, and rounded shoulders are common among people with poor posture. And it is not a coincidence that those same three posture issues are common sources of chest, upper back, and neck pain.

Improving your posture by improving the positions of your chest, upper back, and neck will also enhance the way the entire top half of your body moves. And as an added bonus, your new, enhanced posture will significantly reduce your risk of injury. That is one hefty claim, I know.

REMEMBER

Treating the muscles and fascia of the chest, upper back, and neck does take some creativity. Because many of these muscles are smaller and a little more difficult to find, we tend to focus on zones or areas associated with these body parts. Your game plan still remains the same, so let's have some fun with these treatments.

Demonstrate great posture with marching and squatting between these roller treatments. I love to incorporate exaggerated movements and great postural positions between treatments. This trick is so effective because it re-educates your body to move with a new and enhanced range of motions. For example, if you spent the last four hours with rounded shoulders sitting at your computer, your body will naturally tend to stay in that posture. When you use a roller ball to unlock your chest's pectoralis minor muscle, and immediately march and move with a much-improved posture, it will re-educate your body to maintain this new and enhanced posture.

An Inside Look at the Chest, Upper Back, and Neck

I want you to think about something for a moment. We all know how amazing and complex our brains are when it comes to controlling every aspect of our bodies. The brain is slightly larger than a grapefruit, yet it has almost unlimited power. Meanwhile, every message and command sent to and from the brain travels through the neck. Therefore, it only makes sense that anything we do that puts the neck in a poor position could negatively impact how the brain controls the body.

When it comes to both posture and function, the head, neck, and upper back are all connected. If one of those body parts is in a bad position, the other two are forced into a bad position as well. If one of those body parts is restricted and in pain, the other two parts are forced to compensate, as shown in the following table.

Poor Posture	Compensation
Forward head	Base of neck: Flexed vertebral bones and hyperactive neck extensor muscles
	Top of neck: Hyperextended skull on spine
	Upper back: Rounded
Rounded shoulders	Head: Forward
	Base of neck: Flexed vertebral bones and hyperactive neck extensor muscles
	Top of neck: Hyperextended skull on spine

When I look at someone in the forward-head, flexed-neck, and rounded-shoulder posture, as shown in Figure 19-1, I understand how stressful and taxing that poor posture is on the static and dynamic elements of the upper back and neck. Let me explain.

Unless the person with poor posture is on the International Space Station or the moon, gravity is still pulling them towards the ground. When someone has a forward-head and rounded-shoulder posture, gravity is pulling their head, which typically weighs 11 pounds, directly downward. Simple physics tells us that if a person with poor posture is keeping their head up and their eyes forward, they're winning the hard battle against gravity. But it comes at a cost.

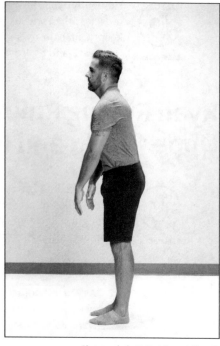

Photography by Haim Ariav and Klara Cu

FIGURE 19-1:
Poor posture with the "bad three" — forward head, flexed neck, and rounded shoulders.

To keep their head up and eyes forward, the muscles on the back side of their neck have to work extremely hard. When their neck is in a healthy postural position, it's mostly vertical and much easier to control by the muscles on the back of the neck.

To demonstrate how much harder your neck muscles need to work with a forward head, I'll use a long rope and a tall tree to demonstrate my point. Envision the long rope tied to the top of a tall, skinny palm tree. If you were holding the other end of that rope, you would represent the muscles on the back of the neck and the upper back. Now envision that tree starting to slowly lean away from you. You are now forced to work a little harder to keep the tree from falling to the ground. Now imagine that a strong wind blows from behind you and the tree suddenly leans away from you another 30 degrees. How much harder are you now forced to work to keep the tree from falling?

With the tree obviously representing your neck/head and the rope representing the muscles on the back of your neck, compare how your neck muscles must feel when you sit at your computer with a forward head for two hours!

Hopefully, you now appreciate how difficult it is for your neck and upper-back muscles when you sit, stand or walk with a forward-head posture. Sit up straight, keep your chin over your ribs, and show your neck and upper back some love! Review Chapter 11 for easy-to-use posture-improving tips.

Ryan Rolling Rules for Chest, Upper Back, and Neck

In Chapter 8, I introduce my five Ryan Rolling Rules. They are my key pillars for my roller treatments. They help you roll effectively, and they keep you safe. I strongly suggest you jump back to Chapter 8 for more details. Following is a brief summary of the five rules:

1. **Align the spine.**

   As you use both the wall and the floor for treating your chest, upper back, and neck, you need to protect your spine with good posture. Maintain a strong spine with an engaged core and chin-back posture at all times while rolling.

2. **Breathe.**

   Oxygen is free, and it's important. Holding your breath while rolling will result in a poor outcome with your roller treatments. Bad breathers are bad rollers — don't be one! Breathing made easy: Inhale and exhale slowly, deeply, and loudly.

3. **Slow roll.**

   While you're breathing slowly, you might as well roll slowly, right? Unlocking a muscle is a timing thing. By rolling slower, you simply provide more time for the muscles to work their magic for positive changes.

4. **Seek and destroy.**

   With the use of the roller or roller ball, your job is to seek out the many painful trigger points in your chest, upper back, and neck. Envision your roller as a military mine sweeper, which drags heavy chains in front of the tank to find and destroy hidden explosive bombs in the soil. Use your roller to do the same in your muscles.

5. **Move the muscle.**

   Level 2 treatments quickly expand the range your muscles and joints will move without pain. The key to this trick is the addition of a specific active movement while the treated muscles are being unlocked by the roller. The details of the joint movement and the roller technique are important for Level 2 treatments, so follow the instructions closely.

Unlocking the Front of Your Chest — The Pecs

The front of the chest is not complicated. The big superficial muscle is the pectoralis major. Covering the entire front of the chest, it's anchored along the sternum in the middle of the chest and spans laterally, anchoring into the upper arm bone. When the pectoralis major contracts, it pulls the arm forward towards your midline. As an example, the pectoralis major muscle is used when doing a push-up. Conversely, when you reach behind you, as when reaching into the back seat of your car, you're *stretching* the strong chest muscles.

PT NOTE

The chest muscle I want to focus on is the smaller pectoralis (or pec) minor. As you can see in Figure 19-2, the pec minor is much smaller and positioned more vertically than the pec major. The pec minor lays under the pec major. It's anchored to the ribs just above and slightly inside the location of the nipple. The pec minor runs mostly vertical and attaches to a bony peninsula of the shoulder blade positioned just under the collar bone.

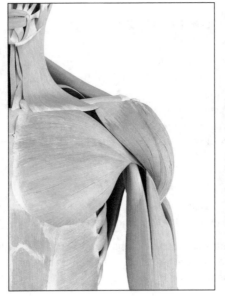
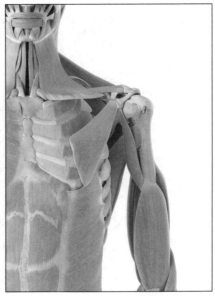

FIGURE 19-2:
The chest muscles are the pectoralis brothers: pec major and pec minor.

SciePro/Shutterstock

The pec minor doesn't serve an important functional role for most of us. So why am I making such a big deal about a small, weak, and functionally unimportant muscle? My answer: The pec minor is a very important muscle to control the movement of the entire shoulder girdle. The shoulder girdle consists of the shoulder blade, the collar bone, and the upper arm bone.

TIP

A tight pec minor acts like an anchor line attached to a boat. If the anchor line is too short, the boat has very little movement as it's pulled towards the bottom of the lake. If your pec minor is too short and tight, your entire shoulder girdle — shoulder blade, collar bone, and arm — is yanked forward, becoming weaker and drastically limited in motion.

Therefore, a major focus of the roller treatments on the chest will involve the pec minor.

Getting ready

As always, perform all roller treatments on a firm wall or padded floor with plenty of safe space to move around. As you prepare to unlock or relax tight muscles, now is a good time to start your slow and deep breathing pattern.

Face a firm and safe wall with feet wide apart and stable. Place a roller at a 45-degree angle on your lower chest muscle, closer to your nipple than your armpit. The starting position for the roller should be low enough so as not to interfere with your head or arm motion, as shown in Figure 19-3.

Before you start any rolling treatment or exercise, it helps to quiet your body and mind. Close your eyes. Visualize your body resting in a relaxed and pain-free place. Perform three slow, deep breaths to prepare your body to heal.

The exercise

Here's how you can relax your pec major and pec minor muscles by unlocking their trigger points.

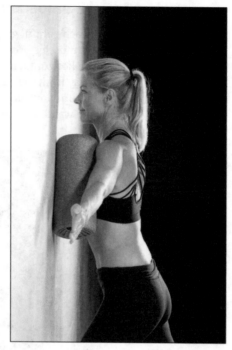

Photography by Haim Ariav and Klara Cu

FIGURE 19-3:
The starting position for rolling the chest against the wall.

1. **Start by slowly lowering yourself down the wall and away from the roller, allowing the roller to glide up and outwards towards the armpit.**

   This is easy to do by bending the knees and using the other arm to guide the motion of your body.

2. **Continue to guide the roller "up and away," searching for trigger points and areas of tightness.**

3. **Continue with loud breathing and slow rolling across the chest muscles until you reach the finish line: your biceps muscle.**

Level 1 unlocking

Rest on each painful grape for three slow breaths, allowing the roller to melt into the muscle like a hot knife through butter. Then resume the upward roll, seeking more trigger points.

If your chest muscles are both looser and pain-free with arm circles and pushups after a minimum of three days of Level 1 unlocking, progress to Level 2 unlocking.

Level 2 unlocking

Rest on each painful grape for three slow breaths, allowing the roller to melt into the chest muscles. Next, keeping your hand positioned approximately six inches below the horizontal level of your shoulder, slowly swing your arm directly backwards away from the wall as far as comfortably possible, as shown in Figure 19-4. Slowly return your hand directly forward to the wall, always keeping your palm facing the wall. Perform this backwards swing two times on each trigger point.

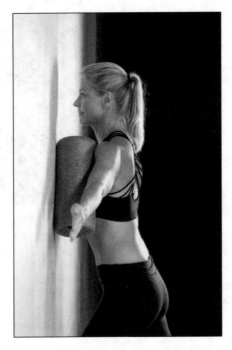 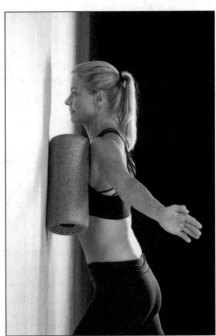

FIGURE 19-4: Level 2 chest treatments involve an active reach back to unlock both the pec major and pec minor.

Photography by Haim Ariav and Klara Cu

Note how much the muscle-unlocking intensity increases when you add shoulder-horizontal extension for the Level 2 treatment. Next, resume your seek-and-destroy mission across the front of your chest, looking for the next painful grape.

Do's and don'ts

Unlocking your two sets of pec muscles is a game changer for anyone with shoulder pain or less-than-ideal posture. These do's and don'ts will help you master the art of chest rolling:

>> Do breathe slowly, deeply, and loudly.

>> Do be creative while you roll — change arm and shoulder positions to alter the length of your pec major and pec minor.

>> Do use a roller ball with sustained pressure throughout the middle of the pec muscle to eliminate any trigger points and restrictions in the pec minor.

>> Do use the floor and a roller ball with jumping jack–like movements to unlock both your pec minor and pec major (see Figure 19-5).

>> Do try other roller options, like vibrating rollers, handheld massagers, massage sticks, and roller balls, to determine the best ways to unlock your pec muscles.

>> Don't roll on bony parts on the front of the shoulder.

>> Don't roll on any area that produces numbness, tingling, shooting pain, or weakness.

FIGURE 19-5:
Alternate
option to
unlock your
pec major and
pec minor with
a roller ball.

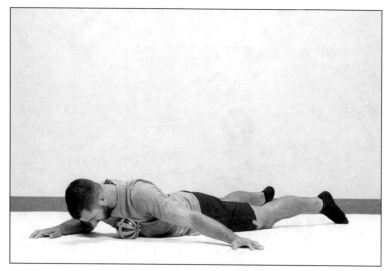

Photography by Haim Ariav and Klara Cu

Unlocking Your Upper Back — Shoulder Blade Stabilizers

The upper back is a big and busy area. It's like the crawl space under your house. They are both filled with a lot of stuff, yet you never really get a good look at it.

I don't want to bore you with medical jargon. I want to keep it simple. I want to focus on the parts of your upper back that have a tendency to be troublemakers. Specifically, I want to focus on the small, but important, muscles that stabilize your shoulder blades.

We have 17 muscles that attach to each of our shoulder blades. That's a lot of muscles attached to a bone that is only about twice the size of the palm of your hand. Many of these muscles become overly weak and overly tight, based on our lifestyle and posture.

The muscles I want to focus on with the roller and rollerball are located on both sides of the thoracic spine between both shoulder blades, as seen in Figure 19-6 below. Because these muscles are small and completely in your blind spot, I want you to experiment using a stretch cord and different arm motions to alter the length of these muscles during the roller treatments. And, as I previously suggested, creatively using different types of rollers, the floor, the wall, and even a sock can drastically enhance your roller treatments.

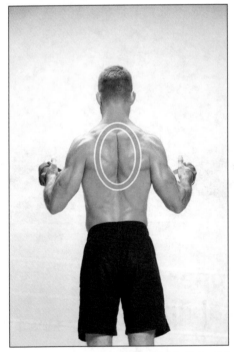

FIGURE 19-6:
Shoulder blade stabilizer muscles located between each shoulder blade and the thoracic spine.

SciePro/Shutterstock

Getting ready

As always, perform all roller treatments on a firmly padded surface with plenty of safe space to move around.

As you prepare to unlock or relax tight muscles, now is a good time to start your slow and deep breathing pattern.

Start by lying on your back on the floor with both legs bent and feet placed wider than your hips. Place a full roller or half roller parallel to your spine. Position the roller high enough to support your head. Most importantly, guide the full roller or half roller slightly to one side of your spine to apply pressure on the muscles just inside the shoulder blade and *not* on the bones of the spine.

Lastly, have a three- to four-foot stretch cord or strap in both hands to assist with mobilizing the shoulder blades, as shown in Figure 19-7.

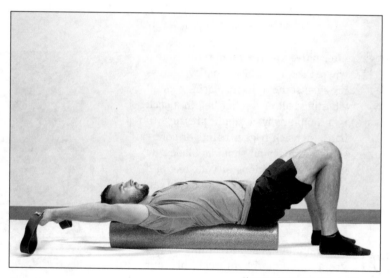

FIGURE 19-7: Rolling the shoulder blade stabilizers.

Photography by Haim Ariav and Klara Cu

Before you start any rolling treatment or exercise, it helps to quiet your body and mind. Close your eyes. Visualize your body resting in a relaxed and pain-free place. Perform three slow, deep breaths to prepare your body to heal.

The exercise

Here's how you can relax your shoulder blade–stabilizing muscles by unlocking their trigger points.

PT NOTE

1. **Start by raising your arms above your head, with the stretch cord in both hands, about shoulder width apart.**

   Arm elevation with the stretch cord is a great way to separate the two shoulder blades and expose their stabilizing muscles and fascia. Wide and strong legs will help to keep you stable on top of the roller.

2. **With the hands in a comfortably elevated position, confirm the roller is still positioned *off to the side of the spine*, not on the spine.**

3. **Slowly perform abdominal crunches to create an up-and-down rocking motion on top of the roller.**

   This motion results in a massage-like feel, up and down the muscles between the spine and the shoulder blade. Treating the other side of the spine requires only a simple shifting of your weight.

PT NOTE

Alternative treatment option: Here's where the sock comes into play. Standing against the wall and placing a small vibrating ball or a roller ball in a sock is a simple way to apply pressure to hard-to-reach trigger points or adhesions between your shoulder blades. By varying the positions of your feet and arms, as shown in Figure 19-8, you can easily control the amount of weight and stretch at the points of pain.

REMEMBER

Maintain loud, deep breathing as you grind through the muscles of your upper back.

Level 1 unlocking

Rest on each painful trigger point for three slow breaths, allowing the roller to melt into the muscles like a hot knife through butter. Then resume the controlled crunches and arm raises, looking for and destroying painful trigger points and areas of tightness.

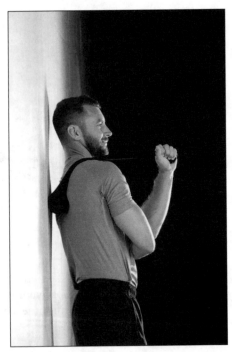

Photography by Haim Ariav and Klara Cu

FIGURE 19-8:
Alternate option: Using a ball in a sock to unlock shoulder blade-stabilizing muscles.

If the muscles between your shoulder blades are both looser and pain-free with arm circles and pushups after a minimum of three days of Level 1 unlocking, progress to Level 2 unlocking.

Level 2 unlocking

Rest on each painful grape for three slow breaths, allowing the full roller or half roller to melt into the shoulder blade stabilizing muscles. Next, slowly pull your arm down and away from the side resting on the roller with the assistance of the stretch cord. Pretend to reach for your front pocket on the opposite side from the roller. While staying strong through the legs and hips to stabilize the lower spine, you can always add an easy crunch to adjust the location of the roller pressure on the mid-back muscles and fascia. Reach to a comfortable position before returning to the starting position. Perform the diagonal crossover stretches two times on each trigger point (see Figure 19-9).

FIGURE 19-9: Level 2 shoulder blade–stabilizing muscle treatments include a crossover stretch to unlock more muscles.

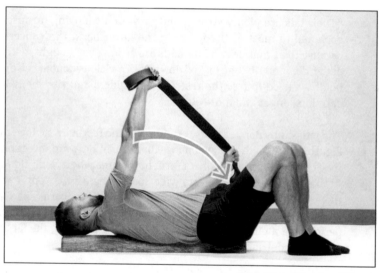

Photography by Haim Ariav and Klara Cu

Do's and don'ts

Rolling a body part on the back side of the ribs completely in your "blind spot" is not easy. The following list will help you to understand what to do and, more importantly, what not to do to effectively unlock your shoulder blade stabilizer muscles:

>> Do breath slowly, deeply, and loudly.

>> Do be creative while you roll. Change arm and torso positions to alter the pressure on the muscles between the shoulder blades.

>> Do try the roller-ball-in-a-sock trick to isolate chronic, painful restrictions.

>> Do try other roller options, like vibrating rollers, handheld massagers, and a massage stick.

>> Don't roll on bony parts of the spine or shoulder blades — roll on soft tissue.

>> Don't be too aggressive with the crossover stretch in the Level 2 treatment.

>> Don't roll on any area that produces numbness, tingling, shooting pain, or weakness.

Unlocking Your Side — Latissimus Dorsi

The scouting report on most peoples' lats would read like this:

"Their lats are plenty strong, and they aren't hurting for fascia because they're anchored to most of the fascia in the lower back. I'm concerned about the lats because their muscles and tendons are so long yet so tight, with their poor shoulder girdles and rib cage locked down with a vicious double nelson wrestling chokehold! We need to free the restricted shoulders and ribs by making both of those darn lats longer and more elastic."

PT NOTE

The latissimus dorsi, or lats, originate in the fascia in the lower back, as shown in Figure 19-10. As they travel up the back in an outward direction heading towards the armpits, the muscle fibers form in the area where your kidneys are positioned. At that point, the lats are very wide and strong. As they approach the back wall of the armpit, the muscle quickly tapers into a tight, cord-like tendon. As you follow the winding direction of this muscle, you can see why it's so important when performing a pull-up. From a hand-hanging position, the lat pulls the elbows in a down-and-back direction.

When the lats are tight and restricted from trigger points and adhesions, which they are very prone to, they round the shoulders and quickly produce a poor posture. Envision a very muscular man with wide lats. Unless he does a great job with his flexibility, the lat muscles will pull the shoulders down and forward, resulting in a poor posture.

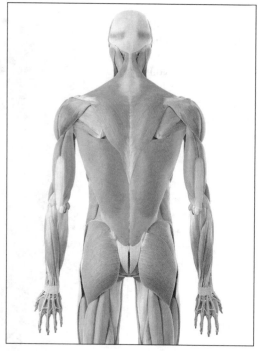

SciePro/Shutterstock

FIGURE 19-10: The long and winding path of the mighty latissimus dorsi.

TIP

Your job with the roller is to lengthen the lats and all of the fascia around the muscle. Remember the track of the lats. This will help you to roll the entire muscle and all of the tendons. It will also help you to realize when you get to Level 2 treatments for the lats, why you will be lifting the arm up and across the top of your head.

Getting ready

As always, perform all roller treatments on a firmly padded surface with plenty of safe space to move around.

As you prepare to unlock or relax tight muscles, now is a good time to start your slow and deep breathing pattern.

Stand next to a firm and safe wall with feet wide apart and stable. Place a roller between you and the wall, positioned halfway between your ribs and your beltline. Keeping your spine straight and your core muscles engaged, raise the arm closest to the wall, placing your palm flat on the wall above your head, as shown in Figure 19-11.

Before you start any rolling treatment or exercise, it helps to quiet your body and mind. Close your eyes. Visualize your body resting in a relaxed and pain-free place. Perform three slow, deep breaths to prepare your body to heal.

The exercise

Here's how you can relax your lat muscles by unlocking their trigger points.

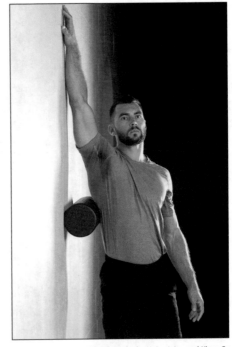

Photography by Haim Ariav and Klara Cu

FIGURE 19-11:
The starting position and path for unlocking the lats with a roller.

PT NOTE

1. **Start by slowly bending your knees, sliding your raised hand down the wall, and allowing the roller to glide upwards towards your armpit.**

   Easy changes in foot positions, trunk rotation, and arm positions will modify the location and intensity of the roll.

2. **Continue to guide the roller "up and around," searching for painful trigger points and adhesions.**

TIP

   Because the lats lie directly on a large number of ribs, the mobility of the lats and the ribs will be similar. If your lats are tight, your rib cage and intercostal muscles between each rib will probably be tight as well. Therefore, the addition of very deep breathing and trunk-side bending is encouraged when rolling lats.

3. **Continue with loud breathing, side bending, and slow rolling, upward from your lower back until you reach the finish line: the top of your armpit.**

Level 1 unlocking

Rest on each painful grape for three slow breaths, allowing the roller to melt into the muscle like a hot knife through butter. Then resume the upward roll, seeking more trigger points.

If your lat muscle is both looser and pain-free with arm circles and jumping jacks after a minimum of three days of Level 1 unlocking, progress to Level 2 unlocking.

Level 2 unlocking

Add a three- to four-foot stretch cord for this Level 2 treatment. Rest on each painful adhesion for three slow breaths, allowing the roller to melt into the lat muscles. Next, with the assistance of the cord, slowly pull the elevated hand up and directly over the top of your head, exhaling fully. Avoid twisting the spine or shoulder. The focus is on swinging the elevated elbow directly away from the wall, as shown in Figure 19-12.

Continue the stretch to a comfortable position, then slowly return your elbow and hand to the wall. Perform this over-the-top stretch two times on each trigger point.

Note how much the muscle-unlocking intensity increases when you add the over-the-top stretch for the Level 2 treatment. Next, resume your seek-and-destroy mission up through your entire lat muscle and all of the tendons, looking for the next painful grape.

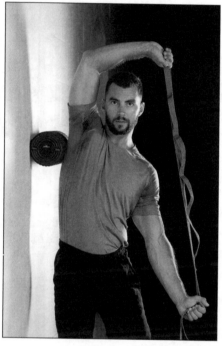

Photography by Haim Ariav and Klara Cu

FIGURE 19-12:
Level 2 lat treatments involve active motion to expand the pain-free motion.

Do's and don'ts

Anytime you grab and pull anything, your lats are engaged. This list of do's and don'ts can help you quickly keep your lats mobile and prepared to work hard:

» Do breathe slowly, deeply, and loudly.

» Do be creative while you roll. Change your arm, torso, and breathing to alter the length of your lats while rolling.

» Do use the floor and a full roller to help apply more pressure to the lats while rolling, as shown in Figure 19-13.

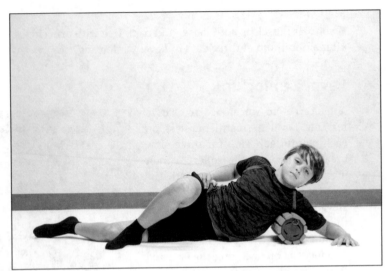

FIGURE 19-13:
Using the floor
and a roller is
another way
to unlock the
upper lat.

Photography by Haim Ariav and Klara Cu

>> Do try other roller options, like vibrating rollers, handheld massagers, massage sticks, and roller balls, to determine the best ways to unlock your lat muscles.

>> Don't apply too much pressure over the kidneys or ribs.

>> Don't roll on any area that produces numbness, tingling, shooting pain, or weakness.

Unlocking Your Neck — Upper Trapezius

The neck has plenty of sensitive tissue, like nerves, blood vessels, glands, and the windpipe, to protect. Be careful where you use a roller ball or handheld device to avoid injuring non-muscle tissue.

PT NOTE

I'll focus on the upper portion of the large trapezius (or trap) muscles covering a majority of the upper back from the skull to the back of the shoulder and down to the lower back. The upper trap, which I will focus on, is the thick, superficial muscle forming the back outside corner of the neck. The trap is named after its trapezoid shape, as shown in Figure 19-14.

The upper trap acts like a strong stabilizer for the base of the neck and the back of the shoulder girdle. Looking back at the poor posture story at the beginning of this chapter, the upper trap would be the major muscle holding the neck and head in an upward position. To bring it full circle, with the example of you working hard to hold the tree up with the rope, *you* would be the upper trap!

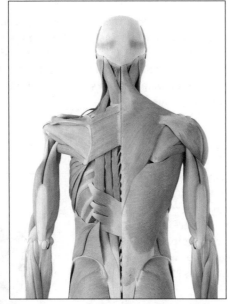

FIGURE 19-14: The upper portion of the large trapezius muscle as seen on the right upper back.

WHY OUR UPPER TRAPS PROBABLY DON'T LIKE US

Our muscles work for us, but they don't have to like us. Based on our lifestyles and common postural errors, we certainly make the lives of our upper traps tough. Here's my list of reasons why our upper traps probably don't like us:

- We do a lot of sitting — on computer, while driving, while reading, and so on.
- We often exhibit a forward head when sitting.
- We rarely do exercises which strengthen the muscles on the front side of our necks.
- We may have poor posture when standing.
- We may have weak core muscles.
- We talk on the phone a lot, with our head tilted to one side.
- We use bad pillows.
- We rarely stretch our upper traps.

The focus of your upper trap roller treatments will be on relaxing the muscle, improving posture, and restoring pain-free neck range of motion. Again, you will need to be creative with your roller ball, handheld device, body positions, and assistive devices. Stay the course, applying the five Ryan Rolling Rules and monitoring for any extreme pain or nerve pain that would indicate that you're putting pressure on the wrong type of tissue.

Getting ready

Position yourself in a seated position, on the floor or in a chair. Place a roller ball on the belly of your upper trap. Use a strap or thick belt to place over the ball, crisscrossing the strap end across your chest and with the ends of the strap held in each hand, as shown in Figure 19-15.

As you prepare to unlock or relax tight muscles, now is a good time to start your slow and deep breathing pattern.

Place yourself in a good postural position: with chin back, shoulders back, and a healthy lumbar sway position.

Before you start any rolling treatment or exercise, it helps to quiet your body and mind. Close your eyes. Visualize your body resting in a relaxed and pain-free place. Perform three slow, deep breaths to prepare your body to heal.

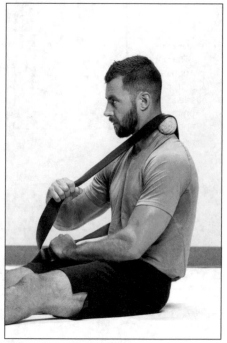

Photography by Haim Ariav and Klara Cu

FIGURE 19-15:
Eliminating trigger points and restrictions in the upper trap.

The exercise

Here's how you can relax your upper trap muscle by unlocking its trigger points.

1. **Start by slowly pulling and shifting both ends of the strap to move the ball around your upper trap muscle.**

    Altering arm, shoulder, and neck positions will help you scan your entire upper trap muscle belly.

2. **Make a strong effort to maintain your chin-back, strong neck posture.**

   You may periodically need to manually move the ball and strap as you change positions.

3. **Continue to apply strong pressure on the many trigger points looming within your upper traps.**

PT NOTE

Alternative treatment option: A vibrating massage gun is my favorite alternative treatment for relieving tightness within my upper traps. Holding it in the hand on the same side as the treatment helps to put the trap in a shortened position and helps the muscle to respond more quickly to the massager, as shown in Figure 19-16.

Level 1 unlocking

Rest on each painful grape for three slow breaths, allowing the roller to melt into the muscle like a hot knife through butter. Then resume the upward roll, seeking more trigger points.

If your upper trap muscle is both looser and pain-free with arm circles and jumping jacks after a minimum of three days of Level 1 unlocking, progress to Level 2 unlocking.

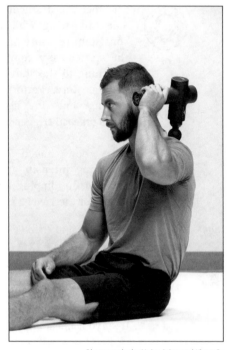

Photography by Haim Ariav and Klara Cu

FIGURE 19-16:
Using a handheld massager on the upper trap.

Level 2 unlocking

Rest on each painful adhesion for three slow breaths, allowing the roller to melt into the upper trap muscle. Next, while maintaining the pressure on the roller ball with the strong band, slowly bend your neck, looking down and away from the roller ball while fully exhaling, as shown in Figure 19-17. This down-and-away movement of the chin is cautiously performed for a comfortable stretch before returning the head to the starting position two times on each trigger point.

With the pressure of the roller ball, this stretch can become intense. Do not overdo this movement! Start slowly with a small movement at first. Progress as tolerable, while never going past a moderate intensity.

The focus is a smooth dipping and side chin-swing. While maintaining a consistent pressure on the ball, keep the stretch very comfortable before returning to the starting position of good posture. Perform the smooth dipping and side chin-swing two times on each trigger point.

Note how much the muscle-unlocking intensity increases when you add the dipping and side chin-swing for the Level 2 treatment.

Do's and don'ts

The neck is filled with lots of important nerves and blood vessels. Follow these do's and don'ts closely to safely treat your neck:

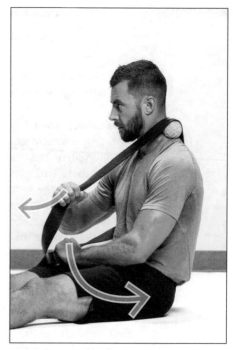

Photography by Haim Ariav and Klara Cu

FIGURE 19-17:
Level 2 upper trap treatment helps to eliminate muscle tension headaches during prolonged sitting.

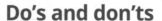

» Do breathe slowly, deeply, and loudly.

» Do only roll the muscles on the back of the neck, not on the side or front of the neck.

» Don't roll on bony parts of the back or front of the neck.

» Don't roll on any area that produces numbness, tingling, shooting pain, or weakness.

elbows, wrists, and hands

» **Unlocking muscles in your shoulders, forearms, and hands with a roller and roller balls**

» **Improving the function of the entire upper extremity to live a more active lifestyle**

Chapter **20**
Unlocking Your Shoulders and Arms

O ur shoulders and arms put us in touch with our environment. Our minds tell us where to go, our eyes show us how to get there, and our legs get us there. But it's our shoulders and arms that reach out to feel and bring our settings into our senses.

With that being said, keeping our highly skilled upper extremity healthy is very important. Anything we pick up, push, or pull becomes part of our upper extremity. The stress and load in contact with our hands is instantly transferred to the muscles and joints in our shoulders and arms. If one of the joints in our fingers, hands, wrists, forearms, elbows, or shoulders is restricted, it puts excess stress on other muscles or joints within our upper extremity. We can't let that happen. I often see this pattern: a restricted joint creating overload elsewhere, causing an overuse injury.

PT NOTE

When it comes to the importance of maintaining high function in our shoulders and arms, it boils down to two reasons:

» **Performance.** Our shoulders and arms do so much for us. Anything we do in our work, in our lives, with our families, and in our sports demands functional and strong shoulders and arms. When we suffer from, say, a shoulder injury, the impact on our lives is significant. Therefore, keeping our shoulders and arms healthy and strong is a high priority for all of us.

>> **Pain.** Our shoulders and arms can be a huge source of pain. Our shoulder joints, for example, are the most mobile joints in our body. Therefore, and when we have a dysfunction of this joint with an extreme amount of motion, it's very debilitating.

Rollers, roller balls, and vibrating rollers are very effective for our shoulders and arms. Restoring motion to both muscles and joints of the upper extremity with rollers is my objective in this chapter.

An Inside Look at the Shoulders and Arms

Mobility is inversely related to stability. In other words, the *more* motion a joint has, the *less* stability it has.

The shoulder joint is the most mobile joint in the human body, but structurally, the shoulder joint is very unstable. Conversely, the hip joint is very stable, but the hip joint has much less motion compared to the shoulder joint. That's why you probably know many people who have dislocated their shoulders, but I'm willing to bet you probably don't know anyone who has dislocated their hip. Mechanically speaking, this is why your very mobile shoulder is great for throwing a ball but not very good for walking on your hands.

PT NOTE

Before you learn about the roller treatments for the upper extremity, note that many of the joints in the upper extremity are controlled by muscles located well above those joints. In other words, a painful trigger point or adhesion in, say, the shoulder region may result in limited motion way down at the elbow or wrist. Looking at the hand and fingers, most of the strong muscles that move them are located much higher in the forearm.

REMEMBER

Applying this fact, as you use your rollers to treat your shoulders and arms, be mindful to look both above and below the trigger points for symptoms and sources of pain.

Starting with the shoulder girdle

The shoulder joint is but one part of the shoulder girdle. The *shoulder girdle* is a combination of three bones:

- » Humerus (arm bone)

- » Scapula (shoulder blade)

- » Clavicle (collar bone)

The top of the humerus is shaped like a ball, and is referred to as the head of your humerus. The convex head of your humerus rests against a slightly concave surface on your shoulder blade, referred to as the glenoid fossa. When you look at the round part of the joint on the arm side compared to the mostly flat surface on the shoulder blade side, it's easy to see why this joint is so unstable.

How does this structurally unstable joint stay in place? The answer is simple: It relies on a strong joint capsule and lots of muscles surrounding the joint. The joint capsule surrounds the joint like a leathery bag. It holds lubricating fluid in the joint like oil in your car engine. The capsule is a combination of strong and slightly stretchy fascia-like tissue.

The many muscles that cross over the shoulder joint add a dynamic stability to this joint. As the shoulder and shoulder girdle change positions, the muscles around the shoulder assist with stability, along with the functional task at hand.

Moving down the arm

The elbow joint is obviously the middle joint between the hand and the shoulder. This joint is actually a combination of three joints involving three bones. The humerus forms the top half of the joint, while the two forearm bones, the larger ulna and the smaller radius, help form two additional joints at the top of the forearm.

The wrist, hand, and fingers are composed of 27 bones. The wrist is a collection of eight bones, the hand has a total of five long bones, one to each finger and thumb, and the fingers have an additional 14 bones. With so many bones, the wrist, hand, and fingers must have many joints, muscles, tendons, and fascia. This is a lot of moving parts with many potential areas for restrictions and pain. It's now your job to keep all these parts moving freely.

Ryan Rolling Rules for Shoulders and Arms

REMEMBER

Take a few minutes to look back at my five Ryan Rolling Rules in Chapter 8. The following rules explain the simple roller treatment steps to help you roll your muscles safely and effectively. (You can also refer to Chapter 8 where I discuss these rules in more detail.)

1. **Align the spine.**

   Proper posture on the roller is a top priority. It's a simple way to protect the spine as you unlock your shoulder and arm muscles.

2. **Breathe.**

   Keep breathing and don't hold your breath while rolling. Poor breathing habits result in a tighten and protective body. Roller Breathing 101 = Inhale and exhale slowly, deeply, and loudly.

3. **Slow roll.**

   Give your body more time for positive changes to occur. Simply move the roller slow and steady. My roller techniques for the tight muscles require a slow and steady roller speed.

4. **Seek and destroy.**

   Trigger points and adhesions make your muscles weak and your joints tight. Use your roller and my protocols to seek and destroy your painful trigger points.

5. **Move the muscle.**

   With my Level 2 treatments, we add movement to your roller treatments. Active movements with your treatment will supercharge the unlocking of your muscles to improve your pain-free movement.

ROLLER PRE- AND POST-TEST

Use this test to help you immediately feel the benefits of rolling your shoulders and arms while evaluating your rolling techniques:

1. **Prior to rolling, perform five large arms circles from the shoulders with each arm.**

2. **With both elbows in full extension, arms horizontal and fingers pointing downward towards the ground, press both palms firmly against the wall.**

3. **After your rolling treatment, repeat steps 1 and 2 and then compare changes in motion, pain, tightness, and strength related to your shoulders and arms asking yourself these questions:**

   - Are my arm muscles looser?

   - Has my shoulder pain-free range of motions increased?

   - Do my arms feel stronger?

Unlocking the Front and Side of the Shoulder — Delts

The deltoid muscles have three parts — anterior, middle, and posterior — that cover the front, side, and back of the shoulder joint, respectively. Their main role is to assist in lifting the arm forward, sideways, and backwards (also respectively). Depending on the position of the arm and shoulder girdle, the upper extremity has many muscles to help the deltoids do their job (see Figure 20-1).

In this section of Chapter 20, I focus on your anterior and middle delts. The third part of your deltoid muscles, the posterior delts, is addressed in the next section of this chapter when we focus on unlocking your posterior shoulder and external rotators.

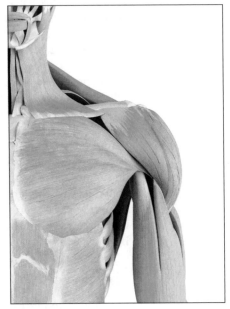

SciePro/Shutterstock

FIGURE 20-1:
A look at the front of the shoulder joint.

OUCH

Roller treatments on the anterior and middle deltoids are fairly simple. One word of caution, though: The upper arm can be quite bony, with sensitive structures throughout. These structures include the biceps tendon and a rotator cuff tendon, both are located on the front side of the shoulder joint. As always, roll carefully and be alert if you feel any symptoms that are extreme or unusual.

Anterior delt

This is where you learn how to perform self-myofascial unlocking techniques on the front side of the shoulder, a common location for shoulder pain. The anterior deltoids cover the front side of each shoulder joint while adding important support to the insertion tendons for your pecs, biceps, and lats.

Getting ready

As always, perform all roller treatments on a firm wall with plenty of safe space to move around.

Face the wall, arm extended outward away from the shoulder, parallel to the ground, with the palm against the wall. Place your feet wide apart and stable. Place a roller, vertically positioned, on the crease where your shoulder meets your chest, as shown in Figure 20-2.

As you prepare to unlock or relax tight muscles, now is a good time to start your slow and deep breathing pattern.

Before you start any rolling treatment or exercise, it helps to quiet your body and mind. Close your eyes. Visualize your body resting in a relaxed and pain-free place. Perform three slow, deep breaths to prepare your body to heal.

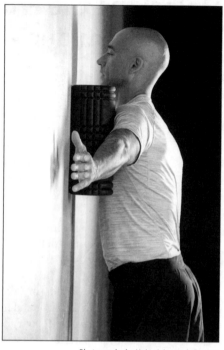

Photography by Haim Ariav and Klara Cu

FIGURE 20-2:
The starting position for unlocking the anterior deltoid muscles.

The exercise

Here's how you can relax your anterior deltoid muscle by unlocking its trigger points:

1. **Start by slowly shifting your body sideways along the wall and away from the roller.**

   This sliding motion allows the roller to glide down your anterior delt muscle towards your elbow.

2. **Continue to guide the roller down the front of your upper arm, searching for trigger points and areas of tightness.**

   The addition of subtle arm rotations during the roll will help expose additional adhesions and trigger points.

3. **Continue with loud breathing and slow rolling down the anterior delt until you reach the finish line: the top of your biceps muscle.**

Middle delt

Strong middle deltoids are widely envied in the fitness world for providing a rounded, muscular appearance to the shoulders. Putting the body building benefits aside, unrestricted middle deltoid muscles assist your rotator cuff every time your lift your arm away from your side. All it takes is one trigger point or tight adhesion in your middle delt to make simple tasks like combing your hair or lifting a weight difficult and painful.

Getting ready

As always, perform all roller treatments on a firm wall with plenty of safe space to move around.

Stand in a semi-squat position next to the wall, with your elbow bent to 90 degrees. Keep your knees bent approximately 45 degrees, while positioning your feet wide apart and stable. Place a horizontal roller at the top tip of your shoulder, as shown in Figure 20-3.

Before you start any rolling treatment or exercise, it helps to quiet your body and mind. Close your eyes. Visualize your body resting in a relaxed and pain-free place. Perform three slow, deep breaths to prepare your body to heal.

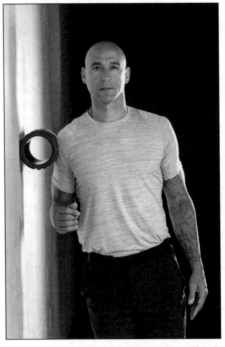

Photography by Haim Ariav and Klara Cu

FIGURE 20-3:
The starting position for unlocking the middle deltoid muscles.

The exercise

Here's how you can relax your middle deltoid muscles by unlocking their trigger points.

1. **From your semi-squatting position, slowly straighten your knees to raise your body upward.**

   Your upward movement allows the roller to glide down the middle deltoid muscle towards your elbow.

2. **Continue to guide the roller downward, searching for painful trigger points and adhesions.**

   The addition of subtle arm rotations during the rolling will help expose additional adhesions and trigger points.

3. **Continue with loud breathing and slow rolling down your upper lateral arm until you reach the finish line: the top of your biceps muscle.**

Level 1 and Level 2 for anterior and middle delts

All my self-myofascial unlocking treatments have a two-level treatment plan. Level 1 involves finding painful trigger points, or "painful grapes," and eliminating them. Level 2 unlocking is more intense and more effective. It involves adding active muscle activation to the opposite side of the roller treatment.

The following Level 1 and 2 unlocking techniques for your anterior and middle deltoid muscles can help you improve the mobility and function of your shoulder joint and shoulder girdle.

Level 1 unlocking

Rest on each painful grape for three slow breaths, allowing the roller to melt into the muscle like a hot knife through butter. After resting on a trigger point, resume the downward roll, seeking more trigger points.

If your delt muscles are both looser and pain-free with arm circles and jumping jacks after a minimum of three days of Level 1 unlocking, progress to Level 2 unlocking.

Level 2 unlocking

Rest on each painful grape for three slow breaths, allowing the roller to melt into the delt muscle. Next, slowly bend your elbow, reaching your thumb towards your shoulder. Bend until the thumb touches the shoulder, or as far as comfortably possible (see Figure 20-4), before returning to the starting position. Perform two elbow bends on each trigger point.

Next, resume your seek-and-destroy mission across the front of your chest, looking for the next painful grape.

Do's and don'ts

"I hope I didn't mess up my rotator cuff" is a common worry for anyone suffering from shoulder joint pain. The following do's and don'ts will help you quiet your anterior and middle deltoid muscles down, allowing you to properly assess the health of your shoulder rotator cuff.

>> Do breathe slowly, deeply, and loudly.

>> Do use a roller ball to "park" on any chronic trigger points with a moderate yet sustained pressure.

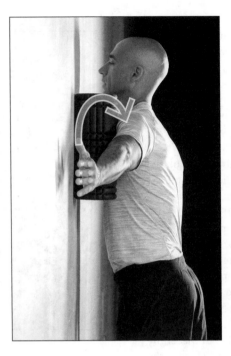
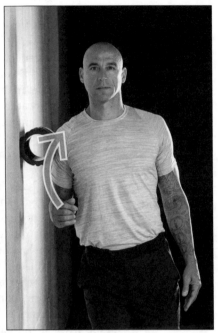

Photography by Haim Ariav and Klara Cu

FIGURE 20-4:
Level 2 deltoid muscle treatment for your anterior deltoids and middle deltoids.

>> Do try other roller options, like vibrating rollers, handheld massagers, massage sticks, and roller balls, to determine the best ways to unlock your delt muscles.

>> Don't roll on bony parts on the front or side of the shoulder.

>> Don't roll on any areas that produce numbness, tingling, shooting pain, or weakness.

Unlocking the Back of the Shoulder — External Rotators

While the front and the side of the shoulder joint are not overly complex, the back corner of the shoulder joint is a much different story. There are a lot of important structures in the back half of the shoulder joint. Each of these muscles, tendons, and nerves can drastically influence both the function and the pain associated with your shoulder.

Needless to say, start slowly. You need to master how you treat this part of your shoulder to keep yourself pain-free and not needing a doctor.

REMEMBER

The main structures in the back of your shoulder joint I want to focus on are your shoulder external rotators. As I discuss in detail regarding your hip external rotators in Chapter 18, knowing the exact location of these shoulder muscles is a must.

PT NOTE

There are two dominant shoulder external rotator muscles: the infraspinatus and teres minor muscles, as shown in Figure 20-5. These two muscles make up 50 percent of the shoulder's four rotator cuff muscles. They originate on the back side of the shoulder blade, and they travel laterally and anchor to the top of the humerus or arm bone. When these muscles contract, as their title suggests, they externally or laterally rotate the arm outward. This is the same motion we use when we backhand a tennis ball or a pesky mosquito.

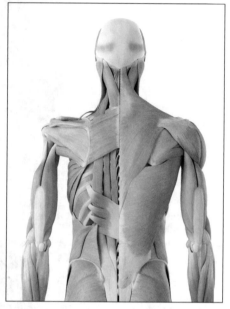

SciePro/Shutterstock

FIGURE 20-5:
The shoulder external rotators, the infraspinatus and teres minor muscles on the left.

REASONS WHY OUR SHOULDER EXTERNAL ROTATORS ARE OFTEN WEAK AND TIGHT

Here is a list of factors which can contribute to your shoulder external rotators being weak and tight:

- Tight fascia

- Trauma or injury

- Excessive tightness of chest pec major and pec minor

- Too much sitting

- Rounded shoulders/poor posture

- Minimal activities involving resisted external rotation

- Congested area on backside of shoulder joint

- Tight shoulder joint and shoulder girdle in an elevated position

My message is simple: You need your infraspinatus and teres minor muscles to be strong and flexible. The strength and flexibility of your two shoulder external rotator muscles is extremely important if you want to be active with a pain-free shoulder joint.

Your roller treatments for the posterior shoulder occur in the zone that I refer to as the *shoulder triangle*, shown in Figure 20-6. Inside the triangle are, you guessed it, your shoulder external rotator muscles. The shoulder triangle is formed with three sides:

>> Posterior deltoid muscles

>> Back armpit wall

>> Bony spine on the shoulder blade

Getting ready

As always, perform all roller treatments on a firm wall with plenty of safe space to move around.

Stand next to the wall with your feet wide apart and stable. Position your shoulders at a slight angle from the wall and raise your arm to a 45-degree angle. Place a roller ball inside your shoulder triangle, as shown in Figure 20-7.

As you prepare to unlock or relax tight muscles, now is a good time to start your slow and deep breathing pattern.

Before you start any rolling treatment or exercise, it helps to quiet your body and mind. Close your eyes. Visualize your body resting in a relaxed and pain-free place. Perform three slow, deep breaths to prepare your body to heal.

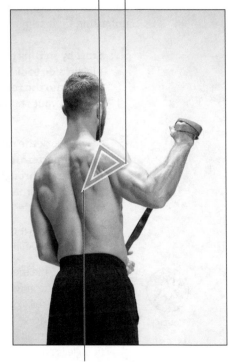

Posterior deltoid muscles

Back armpit wall

Bony spine on the shoulder blade

Photography by Haim Ariav and Klara Cu

FIGURE 20-6:
The shoulder triangle.

The exercise

Here's how you can relax your shoulder external rotator muscles by unlocking their trigger points.

1. **Start by shifting more body weight side to side and up and down onto the roller ball through your shoulder external rotators.**

2. **Slowly work the roller ball in a circular pattern, using the roller ball to scan through your shoulder external rotator muscle bellies.**

    I like to refer to this as "grinding around the shoulder triangle."

OUCH

Personally, the triangle is one of the most uncomfortable parts of my body to roll aggressively. Finding restrictive trigger points and adhesions in the shoulder triangle is easy for me. I'm not bragging, by the way, I'm complaining. The back wall of the armpit is a common location for overly tight fascia with plenty of trigger points.

This is why a roller ball is so effective in the shoulder triangle. The roller ball is small enough to separate the individual muscles and their fibers. Although the infraspinatus and teres minor muscles are the top two muscles you focus on with this treatment, you're still influencing the posterior deltoid muscle, two of the tendons of the triceps muscle, the teres major, and the latissimus dorsi muscle.

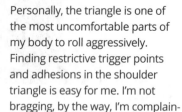

REMEMBER

3. **Maintain loud, deep breathing as you "roll around the shoulder triangle."**

Level 1 unlocking

Rest on each painful grape for three slow breaths, allowing the roller ball to melt into the shoulder triangle muscles like a hot knife through butter. After resting on a trigger point, resume "grinding around the shoulder triangle," seeking additional trigger points and areas of tightness.

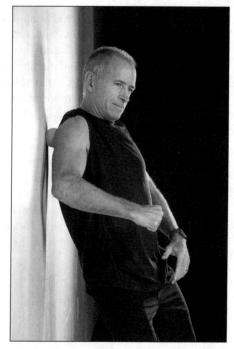

Photography by Haim Ariav and Klara Cu

FIGURE 20-7:
The starting position for unlocking the shoulder external rotator muscles.

If your shoulder external rotator muscles are both looser and pain-free with arm circles and jumping jacks after a minimum of three days of Level 1 unlocking, progress to Level 2 unlocking.

Level 2 unlocking

Rest on each painful grape for three slow breaths, allowing the roller ball to melt into the muscles. Next, keeping your elbow at 90 degrees of flexion, slowly internally rotate your arm, allowing the hand to drop to the floor. This is what I refer to as "closing the gate." Next, rotate the arm upward ("opening the gate"), raising the hand towards the ceiling, as shown in Figure 20-8. Perform "closing the gate" and "opening the gate" two times on each trigger point.

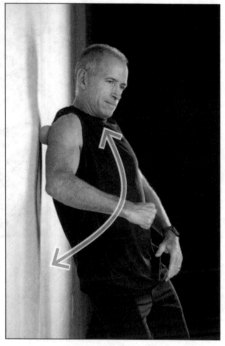

Photography by Haim Ariav and Klara Cu

OUCH

Closing and the opening the gate with a roller ball can be uncomfortable. Therefore, the amount of active internal and external rotation you may have will initially be limited. Start slowly with small motions.

REMEMBER

The more internal rotation your shoulder has, the more flexibility your shoulder external rotators have.

FIGURE 20-8:
Level 2 unlocking for the shoulder external rotator.

Alternative treatment options

Adding manual over-pressure or a resistive band while performing active internal shoulder rotation can accelerate the unlocking of your shoulder external rotators in your shoulder triangle (see Figure 20-9).

Do's and don'ts

If you came out of this section a wee bit confused, you're not alone. Understanding exactly where your "shoulder triangle" is located back in your blind spot and learning how to "open the gate/close the gate" takes a couple of tries to perfect. Think of the following list as a cheat sheet to put you on the Dean's List for mastering your self-myofascial unlocking skills for the all-important shoulder external rotators.

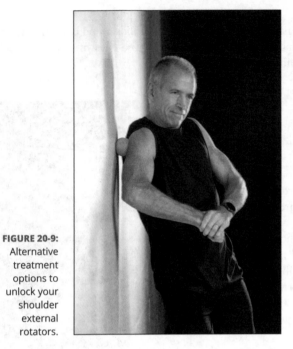

FIGURE 20-9:
Alternative
treatment
options to
unlock your
shoulder
external
rotators.

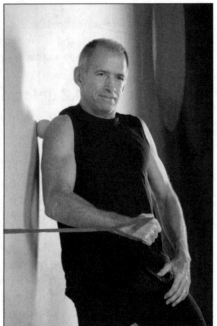

Photography by Haim Ariav and Klara Cu

>> Do breathe slowly, deeply, and loudly.

>> Do appreciate that rolling this body part can leave you feeling "beat up," so start slowly.

>> Do use a roller ball to "park" on any consistent and chronic trigger points with a moderate yet sustained pressure.

>> Do try other roller options, like vibrating rollers, handheld massagers, and massage sticks, to determine the best ways to unlock your shoulder external rotator muscles.

>> Don't roll on bony parts on the back side of the shoulder joint or shoulder blade.

>> Don't roll on any areas that produce numbness, tingling, shooting pain, or weakness.

Unlocking the Palm-Side of the Forearm —Wrist Flexors

The palm-side of the forearm is also called the anterior forearm. It's comprised of eight muscles, most of which travel down to the wrist or fingers. Four of the major muscles originate at the medial epicondyle on the inside ridge of the elbow. The medial epicondyle is a well-defined, bony landmark on the lower inside of the humerus, the upper arm bone.

The medial epicondyle forms the medial wall of the ulnar groove, the trough holding the ulnar nerve on the back inside corner of the elbow, as shown in Figure 20-10. Most of us know the ulnar nerve and groove for its more common name: the funny bone.

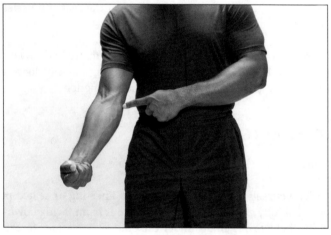

FIGURE 20-10:
The and anterior forearm flexor muscles and the medial epicondyle.

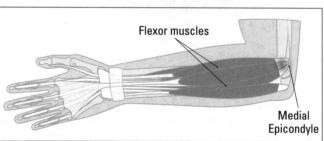

Aksanaku/Shutterstock, Photography by Haim Ariav and Klara Cu

The medial epicondyle is the anchor for four muscles: pronator teres, flexor carpi radialis, palmaris longus, and flexor carpi ulnaris. These four important muscles form the superficial wall of muscle on the palm-side of your forearm. Interestingly, approximately 10 to 20 percent of people do not have a palmaris longus muscle in their forearm.

PT NOTE

The forearm is loaded with tight fascia. Fascia wraps around and through the many muscles, tendons, and joints from the elbow to the tips of the fingers. If you are constantly working with your fingers, hands, and wrists, your upper extremity fascia continues to wind tighter and tighter. Rollers are effective tools to loosen the fascia in your forearms and hands.

OUCH

A tearing of the common flexor tendon, which connects the wrist flexor muscles to the lateral medial epicondyle, is called *golfer's elbow*.

The other five muscles on this side of the forearm are deeper and closer to the two bones of the forearm. The major role of the deeper muscles is associated with finger, wrist, and thumb flexion.

The muscles on the palm-side of the forearm are collectively referred to as the *wrist flexors*. Keeping these eight hardworking muscles loose and trigger point–free improves your grip strength and hand function.

Getting ready

Perform these roller treatments on a stable table.

Position yourself at end of the table in a kneeling or seated position. Place your elbow in a fully extended position with your palm facing downward. Place a roller ball just below your elbow under the palm-side of your forearm. Flex your wrist downwards off the end of the table, with fingers pointing towards the floor, as shown in Figure 20-11.

As you prepare to unlock or relax tight muscles, now is a good time to start your slow and deep breathing pattern.

Before you start any rolling treatment or exercise, it helps to quiet your body and mind. Close your eyes. Visualize your body resting in a relaxed and pain-free place. Perform three slow, deep breaths to prepare your body to heal.

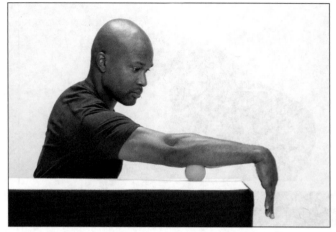

FIGURE 20-11:
Eliminating trigger points and restrictions in the palm-side of the forearm.

Photography by Haim Ariav and Klara Cu

The exercise

Here's how you can relax the muscles on the palm-side of your forearm by unlocking their trigger points.

1. **Place your forearm on top of the roller ball.**

If needed, use your other hand to push down on your forearm to apply more pressure on the roller ball.

2. **Slowly guide your forearm in a circular pattern, using the roller ball to scan through your forearm muscles looking for painful trigger points.**

PT NOTE

Alternative option: By starting with the elbow flexed, as shown in Figure 20-12, you can use the roller ball to apply more pressure on the deeper muscles of the forearm. As just mentioned, start with circular scanning movements to seek and destroy trigger points and adhesions.

3. **Maintain loud, deep breathing as you unlock your forearm muscles.**

REMEMBER

Level 1 unlocking

Rest on each painful trigger point for three slow breaths, allowing the roller ball to melt into the muscles like a hot knife through butter. After resting on a trigger point, resume circular scanning movements, seeking additional trigger points and areas of tightness.

If your forearm muscles are both looser and pain-free with wrist flexion and extension and making a fist after a minimum of three days of Level 1 unlocking, progress to Level 2 unlocking.

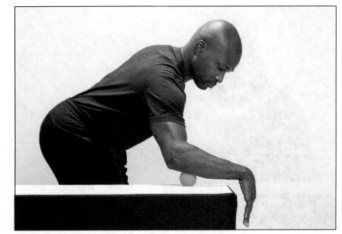

Photography by Haim Ariav and Klara Cu

Level 2 unlocking

Rest on each painful grape for three slow breaths, allowing the roller ball to melt into the forearm muscles. Next, slowly raise your hand upwards towards the ceiling, as shown in Figure 20-13. Continue to extend your wrist upwards for a comfortable stretch before returning to the starting position. Perform wrist extension movements two times on each trigger point.

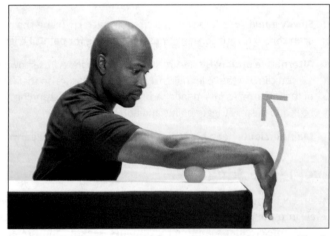

Photography by Haim Ariav and Klara Cu

Do's and don'ts

The palm side of the forearm is the strong side. It's filled with many hard-working muscles associated with grabbing and pulling. Use the following tips to keep your grip strength strong and pain-free.

>> Do breathe slowly, deeply, and loudly.

>> Do use a roller ball to "park" on any consistent and chronic trigger points with a moderate yet sustained pressure.

>> Do alter the positions of your elbow, fingers, and thumb to modify the treatments.

>> Do try other roller options, like vibrating rollers, half rollers, handheld massagers, and massage sticks, to determine the best ways to unlock your forearm muscles.

>> Don't roll on bony parts inside your elbow or wrist.

>> Don't roll on your "funny bone" or any areas that produce numbness, tingling, shooting pain, or weakness.

Unlocking the Back of the Forearm — Wrist Extensors

The back of the forearm is also called the posterior forearm. It's composed of 12 muscles in three layers, mostly stacked on top of each other. Four of the posterior muscles originate at the lateral epicondyle on the outside ridge of the elbow. The lateral epicondyle is a bony landmark on the lower outside of the humerus, the upper arm bone (see Figure 20-14).

The lateral epicondyle is the anchor for four extensor muscles: extensor carpi radialis brevis, extensor digitorum, extensor carpi ulnaris, and extensor digiti minimi. These four important muscles form the superficial wall of muscle on the back side of your forearm.

OUCH

A tearing of the common extensor tendon, which connects the superficial extensor muscles to the lateral epicondyle, is a painful and slow-healing injury referred to as *tennis elbow*.

The additional eight muscles on the back side of the forearm are deeper and closer to the two bones of the forearm. The role of most of those deeper muscles is finger, wrist, and thumb extension.

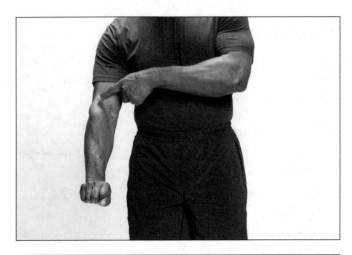

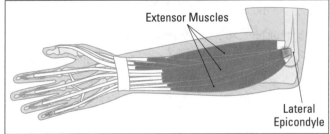

FIGURE 20-14:
The lateral
epicondyle.

REMEMBER

As noted previously, your forearms have a great deal of tight fascia. Fascia is a common source of tightness and restriction in your upper extremity. You know that fascia can synch down on muscles, tendons, and joints. Empowered with new roller insight and protocols, you can treat your hands, wrists, and forearms to keep your fascia loose and non-restrictive.

The muscles on the back side of the forearm are commonly referred to as the "wrist extensors." Keeping these 12 forearm muscles loose and flexible will improve your hands' fine motor control and reduce your risk of injury.

Getting ready

Perform these roller treatments on a stable table.

Position yourself at the end of the table in a kneeling or seated position. Place your elbow in a fully extended position with your palm facing upwards. Place a half roller just below your elbow, under the back of your forearm. Extend your wrist backwards off the end of the table, with fingers reclined towards the floor, as shown in Figure 20-15.

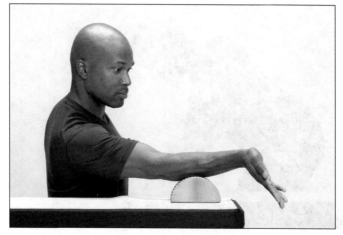

FIGURE 20-15: Eliminating trigger points and restrictions in the back of the forearm.

Photography by Haim Ariav and Klara Cu

As you prepare to unlock or relax tight muscles, now is a good time to start your slow and deep breathing pattern.

Before you start any rolling treatment or exercise, it helps to quiet your body and mind. Close your eyes. Visualize your body resting in a relaxed and pain-free place. Perform three slow, deep breaths to prepare your body to heal.

The exercise

Here's how you can relax the muscles on the back side of your forearm by unlocking their trigger points.

1. **Place the back of your forearm on top of the half roller and roller ball.**

   If needed, use your other hand to push down on your forearm to apply more pressure to the roller ball.

2. **Slowly guide your forearm in a circular pattern with the rounded side of the half roller to scan through your forearm muscles, looking for painful trigger points.**

   If you have thick hair on your forearm, it helps to place a thin shirt or piece of slippery plastic between the half roller or roller ball.

   PT NOTE

   Alternative option: By starting with the elbow flexed, as shown in Figure 20-16, you can use the roller ball to apply more pressure on the deeper muscles of the forearm. As mentioned previously, start with circular scanning movements to seek and destroy trigger points and adhesions.

3. **Maintain loud, deep breathing as you unlock your forearm muscles.**

   REMEMBER

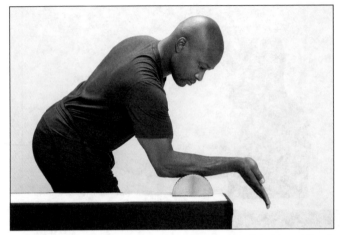

FIGURE 20-16: An alternative treatment to unlocking deeper forearm wrist extensor muscles.

Photography by Haim Ariav and Klara Cu

Level 1 unlocking

Rest on each painful trigger point for three slow breaths, allowing the roller ball to melt into the muscles like a hot knife through butter. After resting on a trigger point, resume circular scanning movements, seeking additional trigger points and areas of tightness.

If your forearm muscles are both looser and pain-free with wrist flexion and extension and making a fist after a minimum of three days of Level 1 unlocking, progress to Level 2 unlocking.

Level 2 unlocking

Rest on each painful grape for three slow breaths, allowing the roller ball to melt into the forearm muscles. Next, slowly raise your hand upwards towards the ceiling, as shown in Figure 20-17. Continue to flex your wrist upwards for a comfortable stretch before returning to the starting position. Perform two wrist flexion movements on each trigger point.

Do's and don'ts

The backside of the forearm is the weak side, so it needs some TLC to reduce your risk of a painful case of tennis elbow. The following list can help you be wise when performing self-myofascial unlocking on the backside of your forearm.

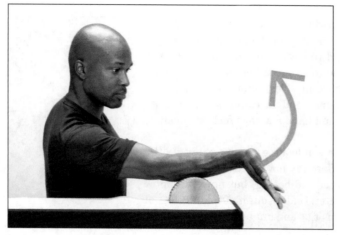

FIGURE 20-17:
Level 2 muscle
treatments on
the back of the
forearm.

Photography by Haim Ariav and Klara Cu

>> Do breathe slow, deep, and loud.

>> Do use a roller ball to "park" on any consistent and chronic trigger points with a moderate yet sustained pressure.

>> Do alter the positions of your elbow, fingers, and thumb to modify the treatments.

>> Do try other roller options, like vibrating rollers, half rollers, handheld massagers, and massage sticks, to determine the best ways to unlock your forearm muscles.

>> Don't roll on bony parts outside your elbow or wrist.

>> Don't roll on any areas that produce numbness, tingling, shooting pain, or weakness.

Unlocking the Palm of the Hand — Finger Flexors

Each of your hands has 27 bones and over 30 muscles to move your fingers and thumbs, as shown in Figure 20-18. Remember all those muscles I talked about within the palm-side of the forearm? Many tendons attached to those same muscles pass directly through the palm of your hand. And when you add thousands of free nerve endings and touch-receptors to work with all those muscles, tendons, joints, ligaments, and fascia, it's no surprise that a hand massage feels so good!

Are you looking at your palms a little differently now? Each palm may look quiet and boring, but now you know better. Under your hand skin is lots of sensitive and important tissue in desperate need of your love.

PT NOTE

Using a roller ball is a simple way to improve the mobility of the muscles, tendons, and fascia in your palm. With many of the tendons passing through the palm attached to muscles originating in the forearm, you can easily alter the length and position of those tendons by simply changing the wrist and elbow positions while rolling.

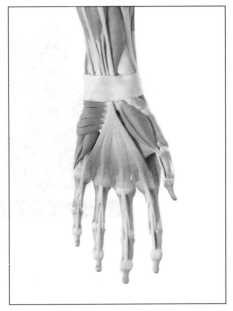

SciePro/Shutterstock

FIGURE 20-18:
The busy palm of the hand.

Getting ready

Perform these roller treatments on a low, stable table.

Position yourself standing at end of the table. Place your elbow in a fully extended position with the palm of your hand facing downwards. Place a roller ball under the palm, with your fingers relaxed and pointing towards the table, as shown in Figure 20-19.

As you prepare to unlock or relax tight muscles, now is a good time to start your slow and deep breathing pattern.

Before you start any rolling treatment or exercise, it helps to quiet your body and mind. Close your eyes. Visualize your body resting in a relaxed and pain-free place. Perform three slow, deep breaths to prepare your body to heal.

The exercise

Here's how you can relax your palm.

1. **Start with your palm resting on top of the roller ball and your fingers relaxed.**

   You will use your other hand to apply additional pressure downward towards the roller ball.

2. **Slowly guide your lower hand in a circular pattern using the roller ball to scan through your entire palm, seeking painful trigger points and adhesions.**

3. **Maintain loud, deep breathing as you unlock your palm.**

REMEMBER

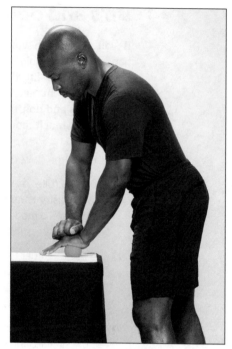

Photography by Haim Ariav and Klara Cu

FIGURE 20-19:
Starting position for rolling the palm of the hand.

Level 1 unlocking

Rest on each painful trigger point for three slow breaths, allowing the roller ball to melt into your palm like a hot knife through butter. After resting on a trigger point, resume circular scanning movements, seeking additional trigger points and areas of tightness.

If your palm feels both looser and pain-free with opening and closing your hand after a minimum of three days of Level 1 unlocking, progress to Level 2 unlocking.

Level 2 unlocking

Rest on each painful grape for three slow breaths, allowing the roller ball to melt into the palm. Next, slowly raise your fingers upwards towards the ceiling, as shown in Figure 20-20. Continue to extend your fingers upwards for a comfortable stretch before returning your fingertips to the table. Perform two finger extension movements on each trigger point.

Do's and don'ts

If you work with your hands, your hands are probably strong. That's the easy part. Using the hand rolling techniques in this section and the following do's and don'ts can make you hand labors much more comfortable.

>> Do breathe slow, deep, and loud.

>> Do use a roller ball to "park" on any consistent and chronic trigger points with a moderate yet sustained pressure.

>> Do use the other hand to assist with finger extension during Level 2 treatments if extra finger flexor stretching is needed.

>> Do alter the positions of your elbow, fingers, and thumb to modify the treatments.

>> Don't roll on bony parts in your palm. Stay on the meat, not the bone.

>> Don't roll on any areas that produce numbness, tingling, shooting pain, or weakness.

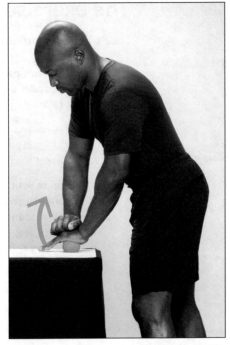

Photography by Haim Ariav and Klara Cu

FIGURE 20-20:
Level 2 palm treatments.

Chapter **21**

Foam Rolling Workouts and Key Stretches

R ollers are awesome for more than just unlocking your muscles and increasing your joint range of motion. I've used my rollers as workout and stretching tools for years. I love the simplicity they provide me as an effective physical therapy tool *and* a butt-kicking workout partner.

Can you name any other fitness or rehab object with such a valuable dual role? I can't.

But I have to admit something to you. The true value of my rollers for strengthening and stretching recently skyrocketed in my mind during the 2020 COVID-19 pandemic. Being housebound with my wife, a fellow multi-Ironman triathlete, and my two extremely active children (ages 12 and 9) forced us to be creative with our workouts. I expanded my roller-based workouts and I was not disappointed.

By now, I hope you know that I'm 100 percent locked-in on physical therapy treatments with rollers, half-rollers, vibrating rollers, roller balls, and handheld massagers. Now it's time for me to share my roller workouts and stretches with you.

TIP

Will these roller workouts and stretches put all the local gyms out of business and force personal trainers to pursue new career options? Nooooooo. The roller workouts and stretches in this chapter will, however, give you a few new tools for your *Stay Healthy Tool Bucket*.

Strengthening with a Roller

PT NOTE

Strengthening muscles and tendons after they've been unlocked is so beneficial. With the muscle and surrounding fascia relaxed after roller treatments, they're perfectly prepared to be safely overloaded with slow, moderate-intensity, full-range exercises.

Forming your strengthening game plan

Each exercise has two workload levels, starting with Level 1 and, when you've sufficiently improved, ramping up to the more intense Level 2 workouts.

Level 1: Two sets of 10 reps; progress as tolerable to four sets of 20 reps with 30 seconds of rest between sets.

Level 2: Two sets of 10 reps; progress as tolerable to four sets of 20 reps with 30 seconds of rest between sets.

Key strengthening tips

These strengthening exercises are challenging and, if done properly, will make you stronger. To ensure your safety and fast results, I want to share five strengthening tips to keep you on track with perfect form with every slow, full range of motion rep.

» Slow and steady movement in both directions.

» Maintain perfect form throughout the exercises.

» Tease the ground or roller with the body part, but don't rest on the ground or roller during an exercise set.

» Add a two-second static hold at both end positions for each rep.

» Try alternative hand and foot positions to vary the workload to help weaker muscles in need of more strength gains.

Stretching with a Roller

Stretching isn't very exciting. I know. I hear you. Most of us would rather spend an extra ten minutes working out instead of using those ten minutes to stretch out. Touché.

REMEMBER

With that being said, we all know how much better we feel after spending five to ten minutes stretching our tired, overworked muscles. And we know stretching helps us maintain our muscle and fascia flexibility after our roller treatments. Lastly, stretching can reduce our risk of injury.

When you look at the value of stretching from those three angles, knowing you want to be more active and injury-free, you'd be foolish not to take five to ten minutes per day to make your muscles longer.

Forming your stretching game plan

Long, stretchy muscles are happy, healthy muscles. Unlike the typical approach to strengthen a muscle, high intensity is not part of this muscle stretching game plan. Here are the seven steps to follow every time you stretch a muscle or muscle group. The consistency built into these steps will help you work *with* your muscles not against them, as discussed in Chapter 8.

1. **Position the body part into a *moderate* stretch position.**

2. **Hold the position — turn into a "stone statue."**

3. **Take five slow, deep, loud breaths.**

4. **Shake out and move the body part.**

5. **Repeat the stretch with slightly more intensity with the same plan: Hold stretch like a stone statue with five slow, deep, loud breaths.**

6. **Switch sides (when performing a single-sided stretch).**

7. **Repeat each stretch two times per muscle group.**

Key stretching tips

Here are your quick tips to stretch properly to improve your flexibility fast:

>> Align the spine and engage the core with each stretch.

>> Never hold your breath.

>> Envision breathing into the muscles and fascia being stretched to help them relax and lengthen.

>> "Listen" to your body to ensure the stretch is applied to the intended muscles, fascia, or body parts.

Upper-Body Roller Workouts and Stretches

Let's get started with the roller workouts and stretches for your upper body from your upper back to your hands. I include your upper back and shoulders as part of your "upper body" because most arm activities transfer the forces proximally to your shoulders and upper torso.

Upper body-strengthening exercises

Try out the exercises in this section when you want a good upper body-strengthening workout using your roller. Each of these five upper body exercises will have two levels of intensity: Level 1 and Level 2. Always start at Level 1 in a slow and controlled manner. Focus on proper technique through a full range of motion.

Many of these exercises have an important balance element included with the strengthening so start slow.

> **Level 1:** Two sets of ten reps; progress as tolerable to four sets of 20 reps with a 30-second rest between sets.

> **Level 2:** Two sets of ten reps; progress as tolerable to four sets of 20 reps with a 30-second rest between sets.

Chest Press

For Level 1 (see Figure 21-1), follow these steps:

1. **Place both hands on a full roller.**
2. **Lower the chest to the roller.**
3. **Return to the starting position.**

When you're ready, move up to Level 2 (see Figure 21-2):

1. **Place both hands on a half roller.**
2. **Lower the chest to the roller.**
3. **Return to the starting position.**

Rows with bands

For Level 1 (see Figure 21-3), follow these steps:

1. **With hands up in front of the body and palms kept apart in a resistive band, lower the elbows towards the floor.**
2. **Return to the starting position.**

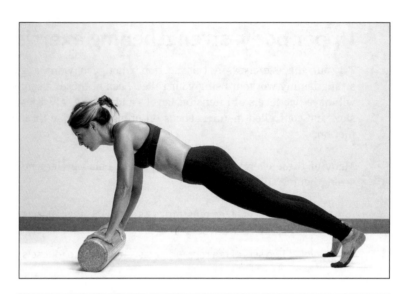

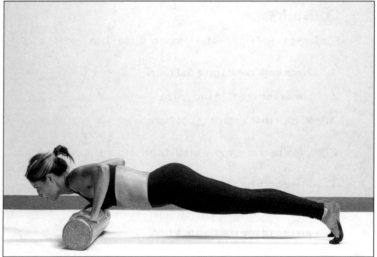

FIGURE 21-1:
Chest press,
Level 1.

Photography by Haim Ariav and Klara Cu

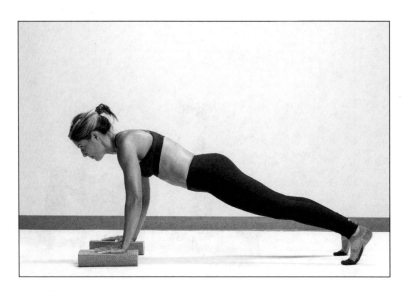

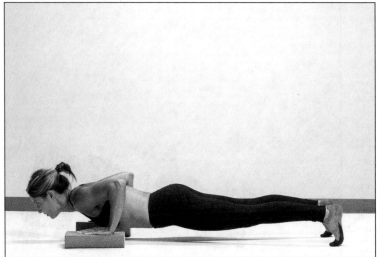

FIGURE 21-2:
Chest press,
Level 2.

Photography by Haim Ariav and Klara Cu

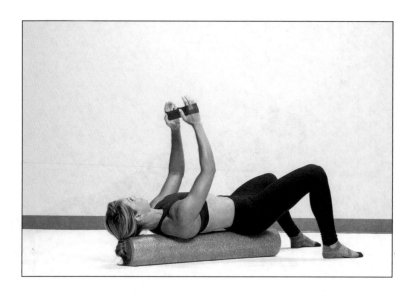

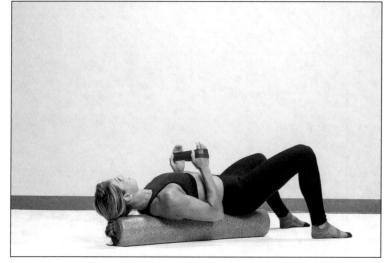

Photography by Haim Ariav and Klara Cu

FIGURE 21-3:
Rows
with bands,
Level 1,
keeping
palms as far
apart from
each other as
possible.

When you're ready, move up to Level 2 (see Figure 21-4):

1. **With hands up in front of the body and grasping a resistive band, lower one elbow towards the floor.**

2. **Return to the starting position.**

3. **Finish all reps on one side before switching sides.**

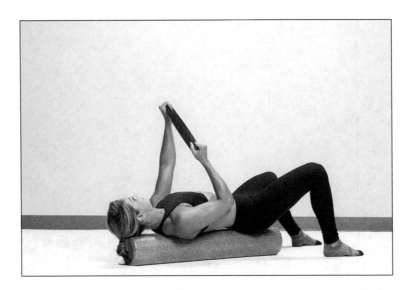

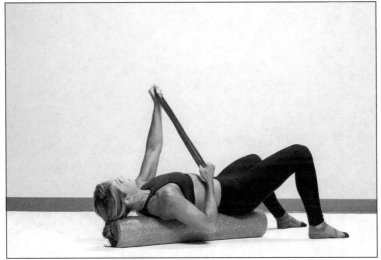

Photography by Haim Ariav and Klara Cu

FIGURE 21-4:
Rows with
bands, Level 2.

Prone reverse flies

For Level 1 (see Figure 21-5), follow these steps:

1. **Lift bent arms off the floor while maintaining a 90-degree angle at the shoulders, a 90-degree angle at the elbows, and forearms parallel to the floor until the elbows are elevated to shoulder level.**

2. **Return to the starting position.**

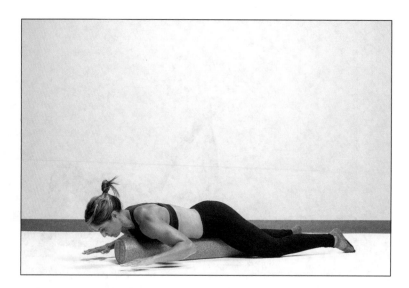

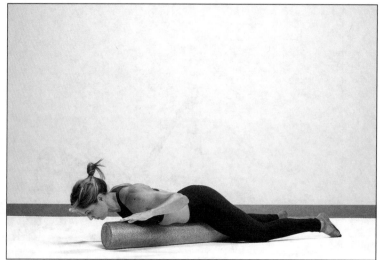

Photography by Haim Ariav and Klara Cu

FIGURE 21-5:
Prone reverse
flies, Level 1.

When you're ready, move up to Level 2 (see Figure 21-6):

1. Lift arms straight backwards, with or without a light weight, off the floor while maintaining a 90-degree angle at the shoulders, a 90-degree angle at the elbows, and forearms parallel to the floor, until the elbows are elevated to shoulder level.

2. Return to the starting position.

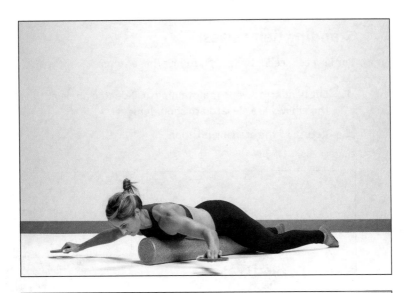

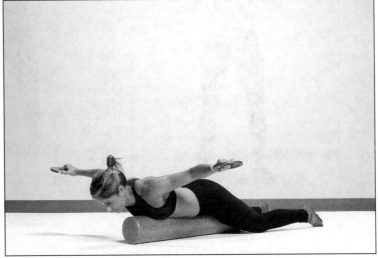

FIGURE 21-6:
Prone reverse
flies, Level 2.

Photography by Haim Ariav and Klara Cu

Standing delt raises

For Level 1 (see Figure 21-7), follow these steps:

1. **Lift bent arms while maintaining a 90-degree angle at the elbows until the elbows are elevated to shoulder level.**

2. **Return to the starting position.**

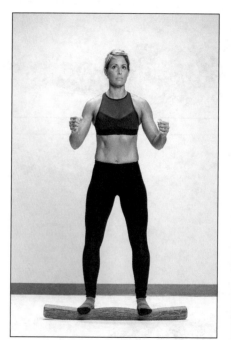

FIGURE 21-7:
Standing delt raises, Level 1.

When you're ready, move up to Level 2 (see Figure 21-8):

1. **Lift straight arms with or without a light weight while maintaining a 90-degree angle at the elbows until the elbows are elevated to shoulder level.**

2. **Return to the starting position.**

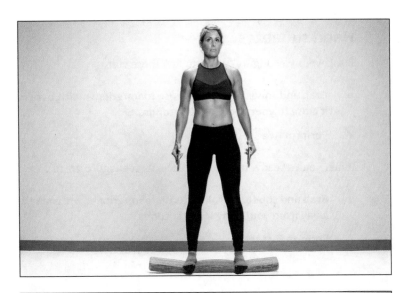

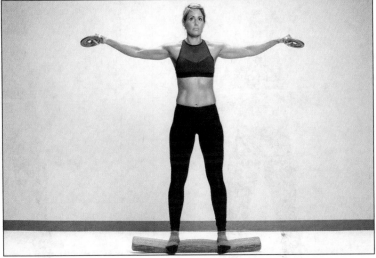

FIGURE 21-8:
Standing delt raises, Level 2.

Photography by Haim Ariav and Klara Cu

Hand squeezes

For Level 1 (see Figure 21-9), follow these steps:

1. **Grab and squeeze a roller/dense foam/gripper with both hands, keeping it close to your body for 30 seconds.**

2. **Perform five sets.**

When you're ready, move up to Level 2 (see Figure 21-10):

1. **Grab and squeeze a roller/dense foam/gripper with one hand extended away from your body for 30 seconds.**

2. **Perform five sets.**

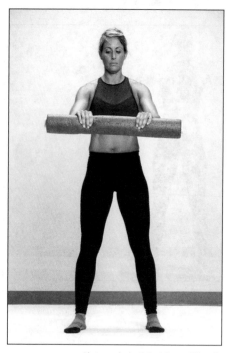

Photography by Haim Ariav and Klara Cu

FIGURE 21-9:
Hand squeezes, Level 1.

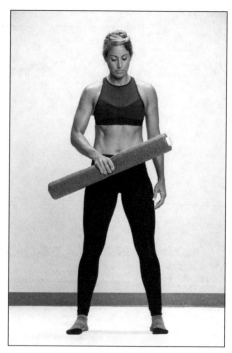

Photography by Haim Ariav and Klara Cu

FIGURE 21-10:
Hand squeezes, Level 2.

Upper-body stretches

All upper-body stretches in this section are performed with a three- to four-foot stretch cord, so make sure you have one handy before you get started.

Review the key stretching tips earlier in this chapter to get the most out of your stretching session.

Lats

With the assistance of a stretch cord, reach your hand up and over the top of your head while side-bending away from the elevated arm (see Figure 21-11).

Triceps

With the assistance of a stretch cord, elevate the elbow towards the sky while pulling the hand toward the floor behind you (see Figure 21-12).

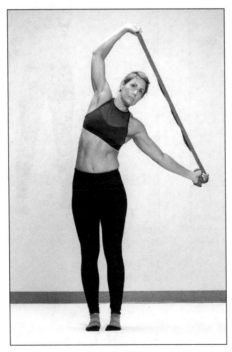

Photography by Haim Ariav and Klara Cu

FIGURE 21-11:
Stretching your lats.

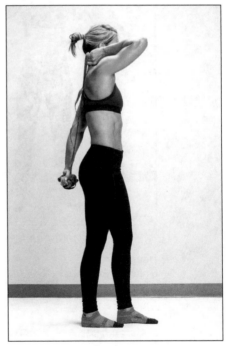

Photography by Haim Ariav and Klara Cu

FIGURE 21-12:
Stretching your triceps.

Chest

With the assistance of a stretch cord, reach the back of the hands towards each other behind your back while guiding the middle of the chest directly forward (see Figure 21-13).

Shoulder joint flexion

With the assistance of a stretch cord, reach your hand forward and up toward the ceiling behind you (see Figure 21-14).

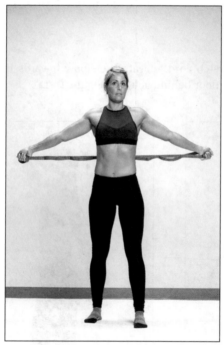

Photography by Haim Ariav and Klara Cu

FIGURE 21-13:
Stretching your chest.

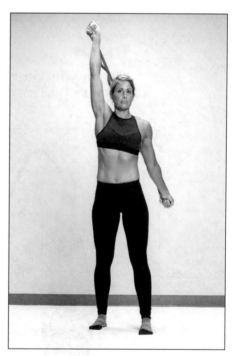

Photography by Haim Ariav and Klara Cu

FIGURE 21-14:
Shoulder joint flexion.

Core and Spine Roller Workouts and Stretches

Your core and spine are involved with almost every move you make. Therefore, performing effective core and spine strengthening and lengthening exercises with the roller is a must for pain-free individuals. The following five strengthening workouts are designed to be very safe for the spine to allow you to be aggressive with your strength work. And when you progress through your Level 1 and Level 2 exercises, being diligent with the reps and rest intervals, your core muscles will be extremely strong, and your spine will be safe and happy!

Core- and spine-strengthening exercises

Try out the exercises in this section when you want a good strengthening workout for your core and spine using your roller.

> **Level 1:** Two sets of ten reps; progress as tolerable to four sets of 20 reps with a 30-second rest between sets.

> **Level 2:** Two sets of ten reps; progress as tolerable to four sets of 20 reps with a 30-second rest between sets.

Crunches

For Level 1 (see Figure 21-15), follow these steps:

1. **With the roller between your knees, chin tucked tightly, and arms firmly anchored on the chest, slowly raise the shoulder blades off the ground as high as possible while fully exhaling.**

2. **Return to the starting position while inhaling.**

When you're ready, move up to Level 2 (see Figure 21-16):

1. **With the roller between your knees, chin tucked tightly, and arms extended skyward with the roller between your hands, slowly raise the shoulder blades off the ground as high as possible while fully exhaling.**

2. **Return to the starting position while inhaling.**

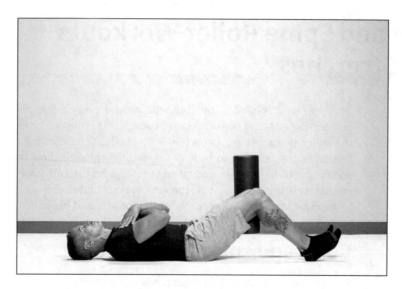

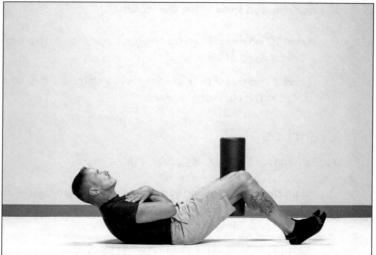

FIGURE 21-15:
Crunches,
Level 1.

Photography by Haim Ariav and Klara Cu

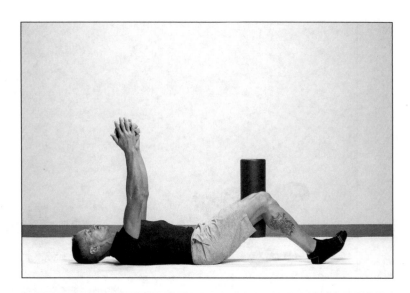

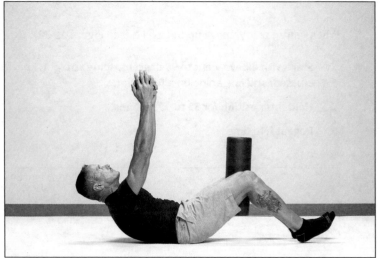

Photography by Haim Ariav and Klara Cu

FIGURE 21-16:
Crunches,
Level 2.

Front planks

For Level 1 (see Figure 21-17), follow these steps:

1. **Start with elbows bent to 90 degrees, spine straight, knees straight, and ankles at 90 degrees on a half roller.**

2. **Hold the position for 30 to 90 seconds.**

3. **Repeat five times.**

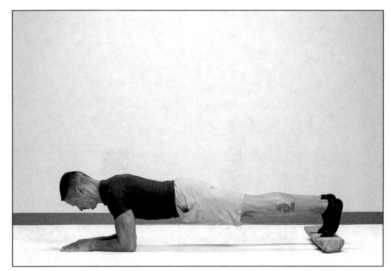

Photography by Haim Ariav and Klara Cu

When you're ready, move up to Level 2 (see Figure 21-18):

1. **Start with elbows bent to 90 degrees, spine straight, knees straight, shins crossed, and one ankle on a full roller.**

2. **Hold this position for 30 to 90 seconds.**

3. **Repeat five times.**

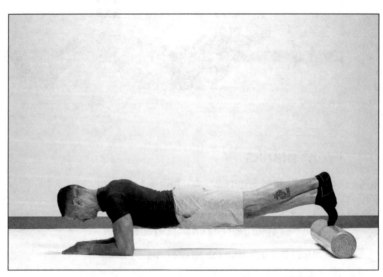

Photography by Haim Ariav and Klara Cu

Side planks

For Level 1 (see Figure 21-19), follow these steps:

1. **Start with elbows bent to 90 degrees, down fingers pointed forward, spine straight, knees straight, and ankles stacked on a half roller.**

2. **Hold this position for 30 to 90 seconds.**

3. **Repeat five times.**

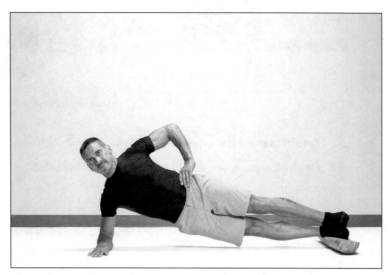

Photography by Haim Ariav and Klara Cu

FIGURE 21-19:
Side planks,
Level 1.

When you're ready, move up to Level 2 (see Figure 21-20):

1. **Start with elbows bent to 90 degrees, down fingers pointed forward, spine straight, knees straight, and ankles stacked on a full roller.**

2. **Hold this position for 30 to 90 seconds.**

3. **Repeat five times.**

Bird dogs

For Level 1 (see Figure 21-21), follow these steps:

1. **Start in the all-4's position with the opposite hand and knee on a half roller.**

2. **Reach forward with the roller-free hand while kicking backwards with the roller-free leg.**

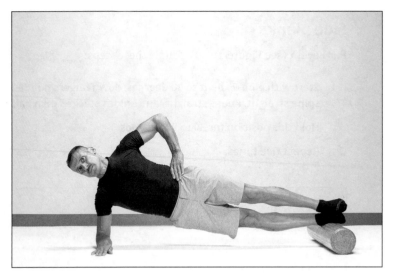

FIGURE 21-20:
Side planks,
Level 2.

Photography by Haim Ariav and Klara Cu

3. **Return to the starting position.**

4. **Finish all reps on one side before switching roller sides.**

When you're ready, move up to Level 2 (see Figure 21-22):

1. **Start in the all-4's position with the opposite hand and knee on a full roller.**

2. **Reach forward with the roller-free hand while kicking backwards with the roller-free leg.**

3. **Return to the starting position.**

4. **Finish all reps on one side before switching roller sides.**

Balance

For Level 1 (see Figure 21-23), follow these steps:

1. **Starting with the roller held overhead, and standing on two half rollers, hold the half double-leg squat position.**

2. **Continue holding this position for 30 to 90 seconds.**

3. **Repeat five times.**

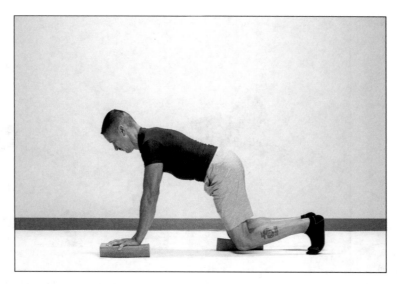

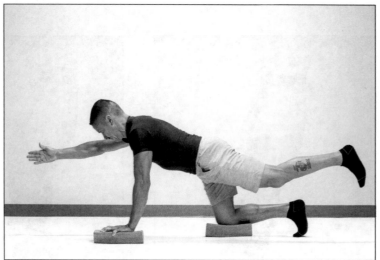

Photography by Haim Ariav and Klara Cu

FIGURE 21-21:
Bird dogs,
Level 1.

When you're ready, move up to Level 2 (see Figure 21-24):

1. **Starting with the roller held overhead, and standing on two half rollers, hold the half single-leg squat position.**

2. **Continue holding this position for 30 to 90 seconds.**

3. **Repeat five times, alternating sides.**

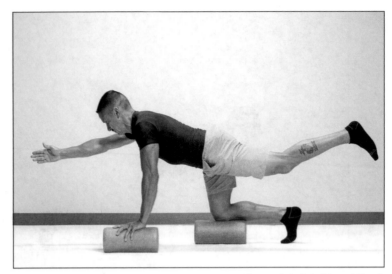

FIGURE 21-22:
Bird dogs,
Level 2.

Photography by Haim Ariav and Klara Cu

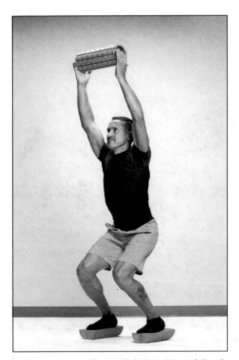

Photography by Haim Ariav and Klara Cu

FIGURE 21-23:
Balance, Level 1.

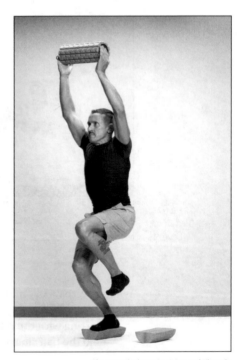

Photography by Haim Ariav and Klara Cu

FIGURE 21-24:
Balance, Level 2.

Core and spine stretches

Having a strong core is important, but having a flexible core and spine is important too. The following four stretches will help you gain mobility of four regions of your spine:

>> Front of your spine with hip flexor stretch

>> Sides of your spine with Lats stretch

>> Back of your spine with low back extensor stretch

>> Top of your spine with chin tucks

I recommend you perform these stretches before and after your workouts to increase and maintain spine and core range of motion. In addition, these four stretches are the perfect pre-bedtime stretches to prepare your spine to recover from a long day of battling gravity and your busy lifestyle.

Hip flexors

Lying on your back with a full roller under the pelvis (not the lower spine), keep one leg fully extended while you pull the bent knee toward the chest (see Figure 21-25).

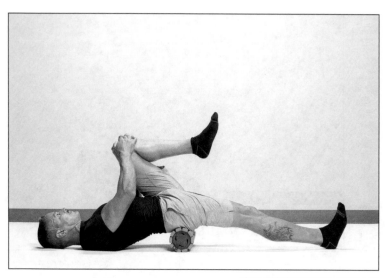

FIGURE 21-25:
Hip flexors.

Photography by Haim Ariav and Klara Cu

Latissimus/groin reach-out stretch

Start in a modified all-4s position with knees wide. Slowly rock the pelvis back towards the heels, glide the hands forward, and let the neck and head melt downward (see Figure 21-26).

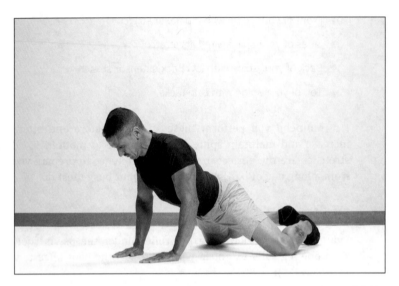

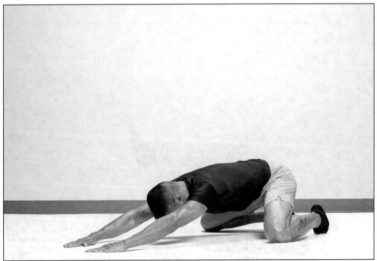

FIGURE 21-26: Latissimus/ groin reach-out stretch.

Photography by Haim Ariav and Klara Cu

Lower back

Start by lying on a half roller with the spine and head supported. Using a stretch band, pull the double-bent knees toward the abdomen (see Figure 21-27).

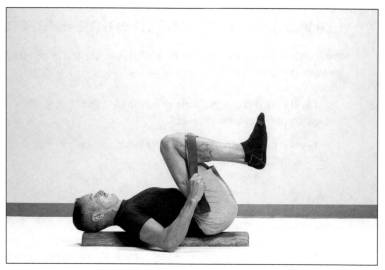

FIGURE 21-27:
Lower back
stretch.

Photography by Haim Ariav and Klara Cu

Chin tucks

Sitting in a strong-posture position, slowly glide your chin straight backwards with the easy assistance of a finger. Hold this position for only five seconds; rest for five seconds; then repeat four more times (see Figure 21-28).

Lower Body Roller Workouts and Stretches

You have so many options available to strengthen and stretch your hips and legs. I want you to give these roller exercises and stretches a solid try for two weeks. What I think you'll find is they're much tougher than you expected, and your legs will be happier.

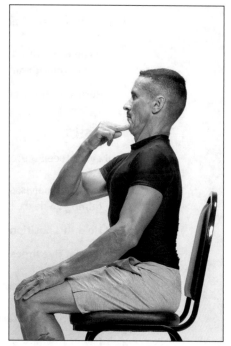

Photography by Haim Ariav and Klara Cu

FIGURE 21-28:
Chin tucks.

Lower body–strengthening exercises

Try out the exercises in this section when you want a good strengthening workout for your lower body.

Level 1: Two sets of ten reps; progress as tolerable to four sets of 20 reps with a 30-second rest between sets.

Level 2: Two sets of ten reps; progress as tolerable to four sets of 20 reps with a 30-second rest between sets.

Squats

For Level 1 (see Figure 21-29), follow these steps:

1. **Standing on a half roller, perform a squat, maintaining a tall spine until the thighs are horizontal.**

2. **Return to the starting position.**

When you're ready, move up to Level 2:

1. **As demonstrated in Figure 21-29 but now stand on a full roller, perform a squat, maintaining a tall spine until the thighs are horizontal.**

2. **Return to the starting position**

Wall sits

For Level 1 (see Figure 21-30), follow these steps:

1. **Press the pelvis, spine, and shoulders against a stable wall while maintaining 90-degree angles at the ankles, knees, and hips.**

2. **Hold this position for 30 to 90 seconds.**

3. **Repeat five times.**

When you're ready, move up to Level 2 (see Figure 21-31):

1. **Position the posterior pelvis against a full roller on a stable wall.**

2. **Lower the hips, allowing the roller to roll upwards until you reach a position of 90-degree angles at the ankles, knees, and hips.**

3. **Hold this position for 30 to 90 seconds before returning to the starting position.**

4. **Repeat five times.**

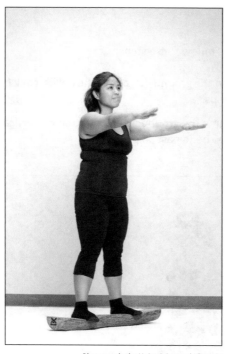

FIGURE 21-29:
Squats, Level 1.

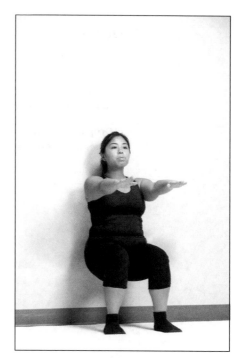

FIGURE 21-30:
Wall sits, Level 1.

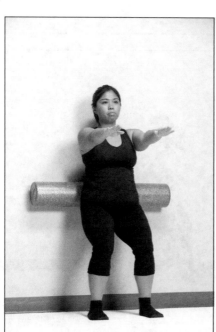

FIGURE 21-31:
Wall sits,
Level 2.

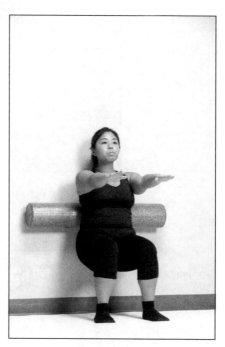

Reverse lunges

For Level 1 (see Figure 21-32), follow these steps:

1. Start with one foot flat on the ground in front of the pelvis, back knee bent, and hands on the hips.

2. Drop the back knee towards the ground, keeping the spine vertical and *never* letting the lead knee bend past 90 degrees.

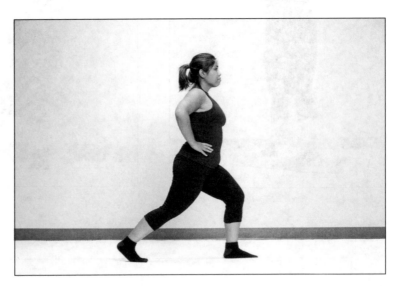

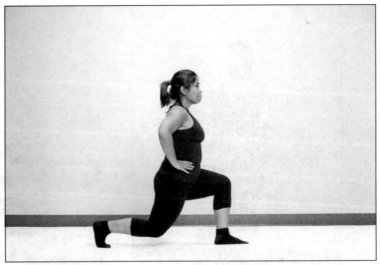

FIGURE 21-32:
Reverse
lunges, Level 1.

Photography by Haim Ariav and Klara Cu

3. **Stop with the back knee slightly off the ground.**

4. **Hold this position for 30 to 90 seconds before returning to the starting position.**

5. **Alternate legs, performing five reps with each leg.**

When you're ready, move up to Level 2 (see Figure 21-33):

1. **Start with one foot resting on a full roller in front of the pelvis, back knee bent, and hands on hips.**

2. **Drop the back knee towards the ground, keeping the spine vertical, and *never* letting the lead knee bend past 90 degrees.**

3. **Stop with the back knee slightly off the ground.**

4. **Hold this position for 30 to 90 seconds before returning to the starting position.**

5. **Alternate legs, performing five reps with each leg.**

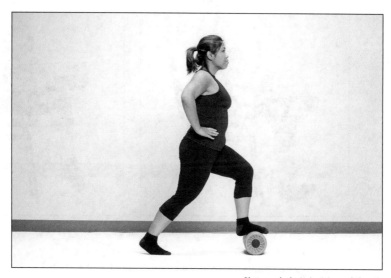

FIGURE 21-33:
Reverse lunges, Level 2.

Photography by Haim Ariav and Klara Cu

Toes raises

For Level 1 (see Figure 21-34), follow these steps:

1. Sit tall in a firm chair, the front of the down foot resting on a half roller, knee bent to 90 degrees, the other leg rotated with the ankle resting on top of the bent down knee, hands on the top ankle.

2. Elevate the lower heel while adding resistance with the hands on the top leg.

3. Finish all reps on one side before switching sides.

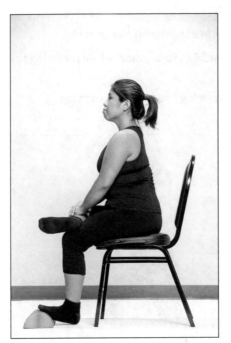 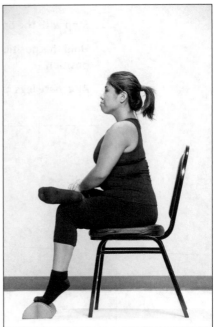

Photography by Haim Ariav and Klara Cu

FIGURE 21-34:
Toes raises,
Level 1.

When you're ready, move up to Level 2 (see Figure 21-35):

1. Standing tall with the front of both feet resting on a half roller, knees straight, and spine vertical.

2. Elevate both heels to raise the head upwards while keeping the knees and hips straight.

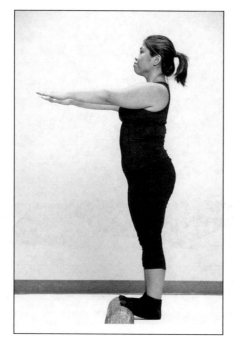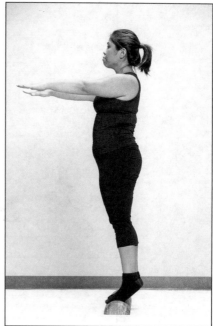

FIGURE 21-35:
Toes raises,
Level 2.

Photography by Haim Ariav and Klara Cu

Bridges

For Level 1 (see Figure 21-36), follow these steps:

1. **Start by lying on your back, legs straight, and heels resting on a full roller.**

2. **Tighten the glutes and hamstrings to raise the pelvis skyward until the hips are level with both the knees and shoulders without bending the knees.**

3. **Hold this position for 30 to 60 seconds.**

4. **Repeat five times.**

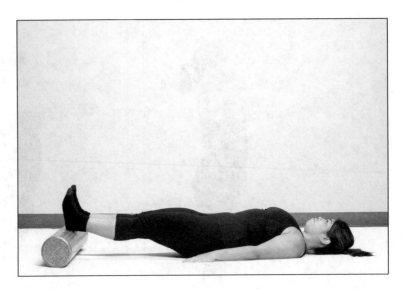

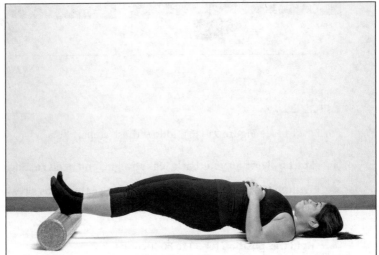

FIGURE 21-36:
Bridges,
Level 1.

Photography by Haim Ariav and Klara Cu

When you're ready, move up to Level 2 (see Figure 21-37):

1. **Start by lying on your back, knees bent to 90 degrees and heels resting on a full roller.**

2. **Tighten the glutes and hamstrings to raise the pelvis skyward until the hips are level with both the knees and shoulders.**

3. **Hold this position for 30 to 60 seconds.**

4. **Repeat five times.**

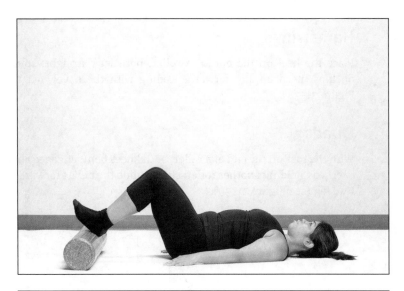

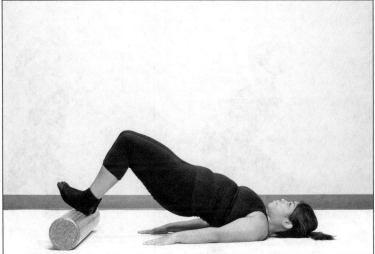

Photography by Haim Ariav and Klara Cu

FIGURE 21-37:
Bridges,
Level 2.

Lower-body stretches

The five stretches in this section help keep the important muscles of your legs limber and able to do their job. Strong legs are great. Strong and flexible legs are much better.

REMEMBER

Be sure to review the key stretching tips earlier in this chapter to get the most out of your stretching session.

Hamstrings

Place the heel on the end of a roller, both legs straight, spine straight, hands on hips, head up and forward, leading with the navel, not the shoulders (see Figure 21-38).

Quads

With the toes on the end of a roller, both knees bent, engaged abdomen, and hands overhead holding another roller, slowly glide the pelvis forward while bending the lead leg (see Figure 21-39).

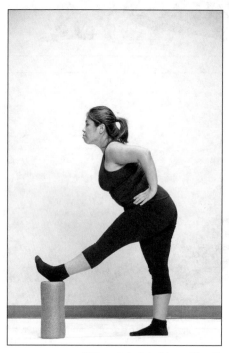

Photography by Haim Ariav and Klara Cu

FIGURE 21-38:
Hamstring stretch.

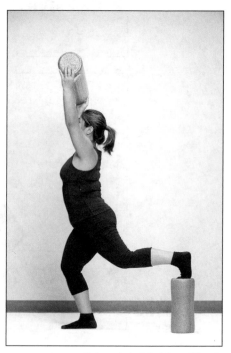

Photography by Haim Ariav and Klara Cu

FIGURE 21-39:
Quad stretch.

Iliotibial band

Start in a standing position, lead leg across the mid-line, and roller held overhead. Side-bend away from the lead leg while pressing the pelvis forward and away from the leaning-roller (see Figure 21-40).

Groin

Start in a standing position, feet spread well apart, a full roller standing behind the bent knee, the other knee straight, and the elbow resting on the roller. Shift your weight towards the roller while sliding the straight leg sideways, away from your body (see Figure 21-41).

Calves

Stand tall with the front of both feet resting on a half roller, knees straight, and spine vertical. Lean forward while keeping the knees and hips straight (see Figure 21-42).

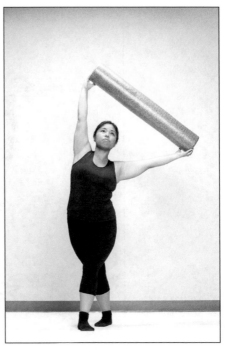

Photography by Haim Ariav and Klara Cu

FIGURE 21-40:
Iliotibial band stretch.

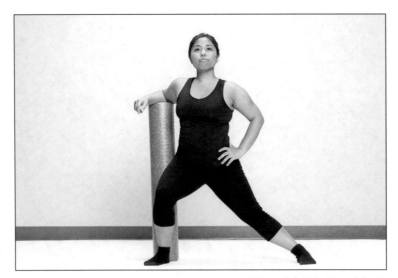

FIGURE 21-41:
Groin stretch.

Photography by Haim Ariav and Klara Cu

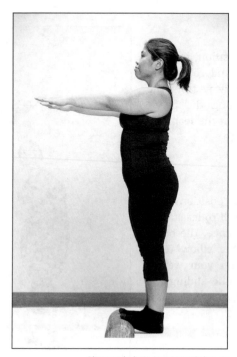

FIGURE 21-42:
Stretching the
calves.

Photography by Haim Ariav and Klara Cu

5

Workouts, Stretches, Injury Management, and Injury Prevention with Rollers

Using roller-based exercises to enhance the strength and length of your muscles

Finding out how to use a treatment planner designed for elite athletes to help you manage your aches and pains quickly and effectively

Matching your sport to specific muscle groups and treatments to stay injury-free

Sports-based body maintenance game plans to keep you active and injury-free

Chapter **22**

Injury Management with Rollers

I f you've worked through previous chapters, you have a better understanding how your muscles and joints function and how roller treatments help repair your major body zones. In this chapter, I will help you apply this valuable sports medicine wisdom to specific injuries.

PT NOTE

I want to help you develop a wellness-oriented mindset enabling you to return to a balanced movement pattern. Your aches and pains will no longer derail your plans of living a injury-free life. By thinking like a sports medicine expert and knowing how to properly use your rollers, you'll have the ability to do the following:

>> Properly assess your body

>> Locate your body restrictions

>> Determine the appropriate roller treatment plan

>> Implement that roller treatment plan

>> Reset your body to move without pain

"I WISH I KNEW ABOUT ROLLERS BEFORE NOW"

I have mixed emotions when, after learning the "magic of the rollers," my patients say, "I wish I knew this stuff six months ago," or "These rollers would have saved me a lot of pain and money the last three years," or "Why wouldn't my doctor or personal trainer teach me to use rollers like this?"

I take great pride in teaching people how to stay healthy. What they do with their new enhanced health is their priority. That is the reason why I pursued a career in healthcare and why I will stay in sports medicine for the rest of my life, Lord willing.

With this being said, and the second half of my earlier "mixed emotions" comment above, it breaks my heart to see individuals with healthy dreams and passions, but their dreams are crushed by a poorly managed injury! When I retired from the Jacksonville Jaguars in February 2014, it was to find ways to help non-professional athletes avoid such disheartening scenarios. At this point in my career, I want to positively impact the lives of thousands of non-professional "athletes" like you instead of only dozens of elite athletes each day.

I know if I can help reduce your muscle and joint pain and improve how you move every day, you'll quickly become a better parent, friend, coworker, son or daughter, and neighbor. That's powerful. And that's why I do what I do.

How would your life and lifestyle improve when you start managing your aches and pains this way? Can you reflect back on a previous injury that would have resolved much differently if you applied the skills from this book?

ROLLER Treatment Planner

I developed this helpful acronym that I use for both my athletes and myself. It's easy to remember and applies to almost any injury or ailment.

PT NOTE

My physical therapy rehab template helps me remove the emotional element of an injury and focus on the purely objective side of the injury. I designed this sports medicine checklist 15 years ago for my injured NFL players to help me stay objective and on-course. I owed this to my patients. I've used this recovery outline with all my patients, including elite NFL players, Olympic athletes, professional golfers, Ironman triathletes, weekend warriors, and everyone in between. It's simple to use, adaptable for patients at all levels of fitness, and, most importantly, it works.

REMEMBER

I ask all my patients to take ownership of their injuries and their recovery. When injured patients take an active role with their recovery and we both work together to get better each day, *that* is where amazing recoveries become magical.

R: Research your muscles and joints (the What)

Message to yourself: "What's not right when I move?"

> **Leg example:** "My hamstring feels tight."
>
> **Back example:** "My back just feels *off*."
>
> **Shoulder example:** "Ever since I woke up in an awkward position yesterday, my right shoulder just hasn't felt right."

O: Origin of your restrictions (the Where)

Message to yourself: "Where do I feel my restrictions?"

> **Leg example:** "It's all coming from the top of my left hammy."
>
> **Back example:** "My lower left back right above my butt is the problem."
>
> **Shoulder example:** "It's a knot right between my shoulder blades."

L: Listen to your body (the Why)

Message to yourself: "Why am I restricted when I move?"

> **Leg example:** "My hamstring is too tight."
>
> **Back example:** "I just feel like the back of my left hip is too weak."
>
> **Shoulder example:** "If I could get rid of that pain between my shoulder blades, I'd be fine."

L: Lay out your treatment plan (the How)

Message to yourself: "How can I help my muscles and joints move better?"

> **Leg example:** "All I need to do is unlock my left hamstring and strengthen my left quads."

Back example: "My treatment plan is to unlock my left hip flexor and hip external rotators while I make my left glutes super-strong."

Shoulder example: "I'll be fine after I unlock my right pec minor and strengthen my upper back muscles."

E: Execute your treatment plan (the Work)

Message to yourself: "This will help my joints move better with less effort."

Leg example: Roller on hamstrings, hamstring stretches, Level 1 wall sits.

Back example: Roller ball on hip flexors and hip external rotators, Level 1 bird dog exercises.

Shoulder example: Roller ball on pec minor, Level 1 prone reverse flies.

R: Reset the way you move (the Reward)

Message to yourself: "*This* is how I want to keep moving!"

Leg examples: Form walking, ankle band drills, half-roller balance drills.

Back examples: Side shuffles, running in place, single-leg squats on a half roller.

Shoulder examples: Arm circles, perfect posture drills, swimming.

PUTTING MY ROLLER TREATMENT PLANNER TO GOOD USE

I used this treatment planner template recently for my most familiar patient: *Me*. I recently did a huge Spartan workout with 20 of my Spartan racer friends. We kind of got out of hand with our workload, and my upper hamstrings on both legs were very stiff and sore for three days. I was religious with my roller maintenance work, stretching, nutrition, rest, icing, and modified workouts. In my mind, I felt very good about my body maintenance plan.

Four days after my Spartan workout, I brought Penny, one of my two rescue dogs, for a run to the ocean beach-club pool near my house in Florida. The run was great. The pool interval workout was great. The fun jump in the ocean with my dog was awesome. And the first 95 percent of my run home was perfect.

With about 200 meters to go until I reached my never-ever-ever-stop-before-the-mailbox finish line, I felt a stabbing pain in my right knee. It was just under my kneecap to the side of my patella tendon. "What was *that*?!" I quickly thought to myself.

I slowed down slightly but kept running (not smart, I know) until I reached my mailbox finish line, clearly in sight and a mere eighth of a mile away.

Walking into my house, I waited for the pain to disappear, just as it had mysteriously arrived. No such luck. Ten minutes later, I was wearing dry clothes and ready for my post-workout routine:

- Rehydrate
- 300- to 500-calorie snack
- 100 Ab crunches
- Lie down to elevate and drain my legs for 5 minutes
- Roll out my legs, back, and shoulders

I added ice to my right knee for my post-workout routine.

Starting the next morning, I implemented my ROLLER Treatment Planner to manage my right knee pain. Here's a summary of my game plan.

Research my muscles and joints: The front of my right knee was tight, and my upper hamstrings on both sides were as tight as they'd been for four or five days since my big Spartan workout.

Origin of my restrictions: The biggest restriction was just *above* my right kneecap and upper hamstring. Meanwhile, my right Achilles was surprisingly much tighter than my left Achilles.

Listen to my body: After an easy ride on my spinner bike and a simple stretch, I took my time just moving. I walked forwards and backwards, side-shuffled, and performed half squats in my backyard, listening hard to my body. What it told me was loud and clear: my stride was too short on the right side. The reasons, according to my body, were coming from both above and below my painful knee. My right hamstring was too tight and my right calf and Achilles needed to be looser.

Lay out my treatment plan: With the body parts in need of healing clearly on my radar, I wrote down my treatment plan on my dry-erase board in my home gym:

- Roller: right hamstring, Level 1
- Roller ball: right calf, Level 1, and right peroneal, Level 1
- Stretch: right hamstring, quads, and calf
- Strengthen: right ankle, dorsi flexors, and calves

(continued)

(continued)

Execute my treatment plan: I got to work performing my treatment plan twice a day, followed by my reward movements (see "Reset the way I move") to re-educate my body on how to move pain-free; then I applied an ice pack for 15 minutes.

Reset the way I move: Form walking for two minutes, downward dog stretches for two minutes, and two sets of body squats, 10 reps each.

My results: My right knee regained full range of motion in two days, it was pain-free with walking in three days, and I returned to running exactly one week after the pain arrived. I added downward dog stretches to my daily routine to keep both my hamstrings and my calves more flexible. I'm happy. Penny's happy, too.

Shoulder Injuries

Your shoulder joints are the most mobile joints in your body, but with that excessive range of motion comes instability. Genetically unstable joints like the shoulder place a high demand on the muscles surrounding the joint.

Managing shoulder injuries is a high priority as we age. To keep our shoulders pain-free, we need to keep surrounding muscles strong, the fascia on the front and underside of the joint mobile, and the joint itself healthy.

TIP

For more details on shoulder self-myofascial unlocking treatments with rollers, refer to Chapter 20. For additional info on shoulder exercises and stretches, bounce back one chapter to Chapter 21.

Impingement syndrome

Symptoms (the What):

>> Pinching and stabbing pain

>> Pain in the mid-range with overhead lifting

>> General arm weakness

Location of symptoms (the Where):

>> Front, side, or deep top of the shoulder

Source of symptoms (the Why):

>> Pinching of supraspinatus tendon in the rotator cuff

>> Pinching the long head of the biceps tendon

>> Subacromial bursa resting above the rotator cuff

Treatments (the How):

>> Roller treatments:

  • Pec minor unlocking – Chapter 19

  • Shoulder external rotators – Chapter 19

  • Anterior deltoids – Chapter 19

  • Lats – Chapter 19

>> Strengthening stretches:

  • Rows with bands – Chapter 21

  • Prone reverse flies – Chapter 21

Reset exercises (the Reward):

>> Resistive shoulder external rotation

>> Rowing with bands, Level 1 – Chapter 21

>> Prone reverse flies – Chapter 21

>> Bent-over rowing

Rotator cuff strain

Symptoms (the What):

>> Lateral shoulder deltoid pain

>> Stabbing pain deep in the front of the shoulder

>> Moderate to severe arm weakness

>> Pain with involved-side sleeping

Location of symptoms (the Where):

>> Front, side, or back of the shoulder

>> Mostly deep into the shoulder

Source of symptoms (the Why):

>> Inflammation or micro-tearing of rotator cuff muscles and tendons: supraspinatus, infraspinatus, subscapularis, and teres minor.

Treatments (the How):

>> Roller treatments:

- Lats – Chapter 19

- Pec minor – Chapter 19

- Upper trap – Chapter 19

>> Strengthening:

- Prone reverse flies – Chapter 21

- Rowing with bands – Chapter 21

- Resistive shoulder external rotations

>> Stretches:

- Lats – Chapter 21

- Chest – Chapter 21

- Shoulder joint — flexion – Chapter 21

Reset exercises (the Reward):

>> Resistive shoulder external rotation

>> Scapular squeezes

>> Bent-over rowing

Elbow Injuries

You certainly don't have to be a tennis player or a golfer to suffer from tennis elbow or golfer's elbow. Those two injuries are covered in this section. Discover all the details about the source of your pain and, most importantly, exactly which roller treatments, strengthening exercises, stretches, and reset exercises to eliminate the pain quickly.

TIP

For more details on elbow self-myofascial unlocking treatments with rollers, refer to Chapter 20. For additional info on elbow exercises and stretches, bounce back one chapter to Chapter 21.

Tennis elbow

Symptoms (the What):

>> Isolated stabbing pain

>> Aching with rest

>> Sharp pain when reaching and grabbing (for example, grabbing milk in the back of the refrigerator)

Location of symptoms (the Where):

>> Outside of the elbow just above the forearm muscle belly

>> Top part of the outer forearm muscle belly

Source of symptoms (the Why):

>> Lateral epicondyle on the distal humerus bone

>> Common extensor tendon

>> Extensor carpi radialis brevis tendon is the most common source

>> Surrounding fascial tissue

Treatments (the How):

>> Roller treatments

- Palm-side forearm – Chapter 20

- When full pain-free wrist and elbow range of motion is achieved, start roller treatments on back side of the forearm – Chapter 20

- Palm of hand – Chapter 20

>> Strengthening

- Hand squeezes – Chapter 21

- When full pain-free wrist and elbow range of motion is achieved, start submaximal resistive wrist extensions – Chapter 21

>> Stretches

- Triceps – Chapter 21

- Back side of the forearm muscle – Chapter 21

Reset exercises (the Reward):

>> Spelling the alphabet with your hand when the elbow is flexed and in full extension

>> Shadow boxing

Golfer's elbow

Symptoms (the What):

>> Isolated, stabbing pain

>> Aching with rest

>> Sharp pain when grabbing and pulling (for example, doing a pull-up or picking up heavy bag)

Location of symptoms (the Where):

>> Inside of the elbow just above the forearm muscle belly

>> Top part of the inner-forearm muscle belly

Source of symptoms (the Why):

>> Medial epicondyle on the distal humerus bone

>> Common flexor tendon

>> Flexorcarpi radialis, flexor carpi ulnaris, flexor digitorum superficialis, or palmaris longus

>> Surrounding fascial tissue

Treatments (the How):

>> Roller treatments

- Back side of the forearm – Chapter 20

- When the full pain-free wrist and elbow range of motion is achieved, start roller treatment on palm-side of the forearm – Chapter 20

- Palm of the hand – Chapter 20

>> Strengthening

- Hand squeezes – Chapter 21

- When the full pain-free wrist and elbow range of motion is achieved, start submaximal resistive wrist flexions – Chapter 21

>> Stretches

- Triceps – Chapter 21

- Palm side of the forearm muscle – Chapter 21

Reset exercises (the Reward):

>> Spelling the alphabet with your hand when the elbow is flexed and in full extension

>> Shadow boxing

Lower Back Injuries

Back pain negatively impacts the lives of more than 70 percent of us sometime in our lives. I want to share proven treatments and exercises that will position you with the happy injury-free 30 percent of our neighbors.

TIP

For more details on lower back self-myofascial unlocking treatments with rollers, refer back to Chapter 18. For additional info on lower back exercises and stretches, bounce back one chapter to Chapter 21.

Lower back pain

Symptoms (the What):

>> Any combination of aching, shooting, or catching pains, or numbness

Location of symptoms (the Where):

>> Lower spine — above, at, or below the beltline

>> Ranges from one side, both sides, or only in the middle of the lower back

>> From isolated at the base of the spine down to the foot

Source of symptoms (the Why):

>> Inflammation, muscles, nerves, fascial tissue, bone, or disc

Treatments (the How):

>> Roller treatments

- Hip flexors – Chapter 18

- Glutes ("the roof") – Chapter 18

- Quads – Chapter 16

- Hip external rotators – Chapter 18

- Lats (the "ladder") – Chapter 19

>> Strengthening

- Crunches – Chapter 21

- Front planks – Chapter 21

- Balance – Chapter 21

>> Stretches

- Hip flexors – Chapter 21

- Lower back – Chapter 21

- Hamstrings – Chapter 21
- Quads – Chapter 21

Reset exercises (the Reward):

- » Form walking
- » Balance drills – Chapter 21
- » Body squats – Chapter 21

Glute pain and tightness

Symptoms (the What):

- » Cramping
- » Tightness
- » Aching
- » Numbness
- » Weakness

Location of symptoms (the Where):

- » Top half of the butt cheek ("the roof")

Source of symptoms (the Why):

- » Gluteus maximus, gluteus medius, or gluteus minimus muscles
- » Sciatic nerve
- » Fascial tissues

Treatments (the How):

- » Roller treatments
  - Hip flexors – Chapter 18
  - Glutes (the "roof") – Chapter 18
  - Hip external rotators (the "ladder") – Chapter 18

- Hamstrings – Chapter 16
- Groin – Chapter 16

» Strengthening

- Bird dogs – Chapter 21
- Side planks – Chapter 21
- Balance – Chapter 21
- Reverse lunges – Chapter 21
- Bridges – Chapter 21

» Stretches

- Hip flexors
- Lower back – Chapter 21
- Hamstrings – Chapter 21
- Iliotibial band (ITB) – Chapter 21
- Groin – Chapter 21

Reset exercises (the Reward):

» High-knee marching

» Swimming

» Body squats – Chapter 21

» Leg swings, front-and-back and side-to-side

Hip Injuries

Unlike your shoulders, your hips are deep and stable. Most of your hip injuries are related to tightness or pain involving muscles around the hip joint. In this section, you'll discover how to unlock tight hip muscles, strengthen the weak muscles, and lengthen the short muscles, all commonly found with hip flexor strains and hip rotator strains/tightness.

TIP

For more details on hip self–myofascial unlocking treatments with rollers, refer back to Chapter 18. For additional info on hip exercises and stretches, bounce back one chapter to Chapter 21.

Hip flexor strain

Symptoms (the What):

>> Tightness

>> Catching

>> Thickness or fullness

>> Weakness

Location of symptoms (the Where):

>> Front of the hip

>> Above, in, or below the inquinal crease (where your thigh meets your abdomen)

Source of symptoms (the Why):

>> Psoas major, illiacus, and psoas minor muscles

>> Rectus femoris muscle

>> Inguinal bursa

>> Anterior hip capsule and surrounding fascia

Treatments (the How):

>> Roller treatments
   ● Quads – Chapter 16
   ● ITB – Chapter 16
   ● Hip flexor – Chapter 18
   ● Glutes (the "roof") – Chapter 18
   ● Hip external rotators (the "ladder") – Chapter 18

>> Strengthening
   ● Squats – Chapter 21
   ● Wall sits – Chapter 21
   ● Reverse lunges – Chapter 21

>> Stretches

- Quads – Chapter 21

- Hip flexors – Chapter 21

- ITB – Chapter 21

- Groin – Chapter 21

Reset exercises (the Reward):

>> Bike riding

>> Swimming

>> Body squats – Chapter 21

>> Leg swings, front-and-back and side-to-side

Hip rotator strain and tightness

Symptoms (the What):

>> Cramping

>> Tightness

>> Aching

>> Numbness

>> Weakness

Location of symptoms (the Where):

>> Behind and slightly below the side "hip bone"

Source of symptoms (the Why):

>> Piriformis, gemellus superior, gemellus inferior, obturator internus, obturator externus, or quadratus femoris muscles

>> Sciatic nerve

>> Surrounding fascia

>> Greater trochanter bursa

Treatments (the How):

» Roller treatments

- Hip external rotators (the "ladder") – Chapter 18
- Groin – Chapter 16
- Quads – Chapter 16
- ITB – Chapter 16
- Calf – Chapter 17

» Strengthening

- Bridges – Chapter 21
- Reverse lunges – Chapter 21
- Squats – Chapter 21
- Wall sits – Chapter 21
- Bird dogs – Chapter 21

» Stretches

- ITB – Chapter 21
- Quads – Chapter 21
- Hamstrings – Chapter 21
- Groin – Chapter 21

Reset exercises (the Reward):

» Jump rope

» Bike riding

» Swimming

» Leg swings, side-to-side

Thigh Injuries

Your thigh has four sides: front, back, and two sides. We will focus on the hard-working muscles in the front (quadriceps) and back (hamstring). The quads have four muscles, while the hamstrings are composed of three muscles.

This section of your injury management plan will help you accelerate the healing of these muscles when they aren't able to do their job. An important tip to share: All of these muscles are long so remember to apply these treatment techniques to the entire length of the muscles.

For more details on thigh self-myofascial unlocking treatments with rollers, refer back to Chapter 16. For additional info on thigh exercises and stretches, bounce back one chapter to Chapter 21.

Quadriceps strain

Symptoms (the What):

>> Localized pain with running and squatting

>> Tightness

>> Aching

>> Weakness

Location of symptoms (the Where):

>> Anywhere on the anterior and lateral thigh, from the kneecap up to the inguinal crease (where the thigh meets the abdomen)

Source of symptoms (the Why):

>> Quadriceps muscles: rectus femoris, vastus lateralis, vastus intermedialis, and vastus medialis

>> Sartorius muscle

>> Fascia encompassing each muscle of the thigh

Treatments (the How):

>> Roller treatments

- Quads – Chapter 16

- Calf – Chapter 17

- ITB – Chapter 16

- Hip flexors – Chapter 18

>> Strengthening

- Squats – Chapter 21
- Wall sits – Chapter 21
- Reverse lunges – Chapter 21

>> Stretches

- Quads – Chapter 21
- Hamstrings – Chapter 21
- ITB – Chapter 21
- Groin – Chapter 21
- Hip flexors – Chapter 21

Reset exercises (the Reward):

>> Pool walking

>> Bike riding

>> Swimming

>> Backwards walking

Hamstring strain

Symptoms (the What):

>> Localized pain with fast walking, quick starts, and reaching for the toes with the knees straight

>> Tightness

>> Aching

>> Weakness with the curling knee

Location of symptoms (the Where):

>> Posterior of the thigh between the knee and the base of the glutes

Source of symptoms (the Why):

>> Hamstring muscles — biceps femoris, semimembranosus, and semitendono-sis muscles

>> Fascia around the hamstring muscles

Treatments (the How):

>> Roller treatments

- Hamstring – Chapter 16
- ITB – Chapter 16
- Calf – Chapter 17
- Quads – Chapter 16

>> Strengthening

- Bridges – Chapter 21
- Reverse lunges – Chapter 21
- Bird dogs – Chapter 21

>> Stretches

- Hamstrings – Chapter 21
- Calf – Chapter 21
- Quads – Chapter 21
- Hip flexors – Chapter 21

Reset exercises (the Reward):

>> Stair climbing

>> Bike riding

>> Swimming

>> Slow jogging

Knee Injuries

Knee injuries are too common at all levels of fitness. With the high number of painful knees comes great confusion related to the source of the pain. This section will help you gain clarity understanding your knee injury and the best plan to put your knee pain in your rearview mirror.

TIP

For more details on knee self-myofascial unlocking treatments with rollers, refer back to Chapter 16. For additional info on knee exercises and stretches, bounce back one chapter to Chapter 21.

Patella tendonitis

Symptoms (the What):

>> Localized pain

>> Deep aching

Location of symptoms (the Where):

>> Bottom tip of the kneecap

>> Between the bottom of the kneecap and the upper shin bone

Source of symptoms (the Why):

>> Connection between the bottom of the kneecap and the patella tendon

>> Patella tendon

>> Connection between the bottom of the patella tendon and the upper shin bone

>> Fascia around the tendon and the infrapatellar fat pad

Treatments (the How):

>> Roller treatments

  • Quads – Chapter 16

  • ITB – Chapter 16

- Calf – Chapter 17
- Ankle dorsi flexors – Chapter 17

» Strengthening

- Wall sits – Chapter 21
- Squats – Chapter 21
- Front planks – Chapter 21

» Stretches

- Quads – Chapter 21
- ITB – Chapter 21
- Hamstrings – Chapter 21
- Hip flexors – Chapter 21

Reset exercises (the Reward):

» Pool walking

» Bike riding

» Swimming

» Backwards walking

Chondromalacia

Symptoms (the What):

» General ache

» Grinding and catching with squats and stairs

» Mild to moderate knee swelling

» Mild to moderate increase in knee joint warmth

Location of symptoms (the Where):

» Behind the kneecap

» Front half of the knee joint

Source of symptoms (the Why):

» Articular cartilage behind the kneecap

» Articular cartilage on the end of the femur (thigh bone)

» Joint effusion (swelling)

Treatments (the How):

» Roller treatments

- ITB – Chapter 16
- Quads – Chapter 16
- Calf – Chapter 17
- Ankle dorsi flexors – Chapter 17

» Strengthening

- Wall sits – Chapter 21
- Squats – Chapter 21
- Front planks – Chapter 21

» Stretches

- ITB – Chapter 21
- Quads – Chapter 21
- Hamstrings – Chapter 21
- Hip flexors – Chapter 21

Reset exercises (the Reward):

» Bike riding

» Swimming

» Elliptical trainer

Ankle Injuries

Our ankles are our base of support. Keeping our ankles limber and pain-free is important for both life and sports. Managing an arthritic or tight ankle is different than treating a case of chronic Achilles tendonitis. I'll share with you tips to manage both type of injuries in this section.

TIP

For more details on ankle self-myofascial unlocking treatments with rollers, refer back to Chapter 17. For additional info on ankle exercises and stretches, bounce back one chapter to Chapter 21.

Ankle arthritis and tightness

Symptoms (the What):

>> Deep aching

>> Pressure or tightness

>> Pinching or catching

Location of symptoms (the Where):

>> Anywhere in or around the ankle joint — the front, sides, and back

>> Base of the Achilles tendon

>> Front of the lower shin

Source of symptoms (the Why):

>> Articular cartilage on the bottom of the tibia or fibula; shin bones

>> Articular cartilage on the top talus bone

>> Ankle joint capsule, fascia, or ligaments

Treatments (the How):

>> Roller treatments

- Ankle dorsi flexors – Chapter 17

- Calf – Chapter 17

- Peroneals – Chapter 17
- Arch – Chapter 17

» Strengthening

- Toe raises – Chapter 21
- Balance drills – Chapter 21
- Duck walks

» Stretches

- Calves – Chapter 21
- Quads – Chapter 21

Reset exercises (the Reward):

» Form walking

» Balance drills – Chapter 21

» Bent-knee side shuffles

Achilles tendonitis

Symptoms (the What):

» Stabbing pain

» Aching with running, and climbing stairs and hills

» Mild to moderate tightness

Location of symptoms (the Where):

» In or around the Achilles tendon from the base of the calf muscles to the heel bone

Source of symptoms (the Why):

» Achilles tendon

» Sheath and fascia around the Achilles tendon

Treatments (the How):

- **»** Roller treatments
  - Peroneals – Chapter 17
  - Calves – Chapter 17
  - Ankle dorsi flexors – Chapter 17
  - Arch – Chapter 17
- **»** Strengthening
  - Squats – Chapter 21
  - Toe raises – Chapter 21
  - Reverse lunges – Chapter 21
- **»** Stretches
  - Calves – Chapter 21
  - Hamstrings – Chapter 21

Reset exercises (the Reward):

- **»** Body squat, keeping the heels down – Chapter 21
- **»** Form walking
- **»** Balance drills – Chapter 21

SPORTS MEDICINE TIPS

I love sports medicine. It provides helpful advice to keep people, not just athletes, healthy and active. Here are a few of my favorite sports medicine tips:

- "Motion is Lotion": Movement keeps your muscles, tendons, joints, ligaments, fascia, skin, and articular cartilage healthier.
- Don't go it alone: Seek the advice of experts.
- Ice is your best friend: If it's swollen, warm, sore, or red, ice it!
- Think HEALTHY: Drink more water, eat healthy, stretch more, and sleep more.
- Work on your balance: Regardless of your age, better balance is a huge advantage for your body, brain, lifestyle, and safety.

Chapter **23**

Injury Prevention with Rollers for Your Sports

Y ou now have the tools, the techniques, the treatments, the injury management, and the mindset to keep your muscles and joints moving as you intend them to move. Now it's time to apply the magic of the rollers to prevent injuries.

REMEMBER

It only seems logical. If you know rollers are great at unlocking muscles, mobilizing fascia, warming up soft tissue, increasing joint range of motion, and improving how your body moves, why wouldn't you apply that sports medicine wisdom to *prevent* injuries?

What Is Injury Prevention?

Many of us have that one sport or activity that we love to do. Everything about the sport seems to blend with us as a person. We're comfortable with it. It mixes well with our schedule and our friends. In a crazy kind of way, our sports "gets" us.

We consistently use our one primary sport for many reasons:

>> Stress management

>> Weight reduction

>> Strength training

>> Socializing

>> Social media posts

>> Time away from work, kids, in-laws, finances, homework, home projects, To-Do lists, and so on

>> Adventure

>> Creative thinking

PT NOTE

All those reasons are perfect motivators to get out and move. But there's one problem: Using one sport or activity so often, for so long, and for so many reasons has a very strong tendency to alter the muscle balance in your body. Stronger muscles get stronger and tighter, while the weaker muscles get weaker and longer.

It's the perfect formula for an overuse injury.

In addition, when a muscle imbalance gets worse over time, a person's posture demonstrates those imbalances. Have you noticed how you can tell a person's sport by the way they stand and walk? They just seem to have the "look" of a runner or basketball player or CrossFitter. What you're seeing is a muscle imbalance in their posture.

I'm taking the long, scenic route to answer the question posed in the title of this section, "What is Injury Prevention?"

Again, keeping to my quest to keep things simple, I define *injury prevention* as follows: *Injury prevention is the act of reducing the risk and/or severity of bodily harm.*

Some might say, "Well if they still get injured, they must have done a poor job with their injury prevention." I don't agree. If we wanted to prevent all injuries for a person, we'd bubble-wrap them, lock them in a padded room, and implement 100 percent abstinence. That'd certainly be injury prevention overkill.

Instead, I focus on smart injury prevention both *above* the neck and *below* it. In other words, I educate the person on the science of preventing injuries and help them perform specific exercises and stretches, based on their sport or activity, to keep their muscles balanced.

As I discuss in Chapter 12, keeping muscles on both sides of the joints and on both sides of the body balanced keeps the body functioning well. A muscle imbalance, like a misaligned car tire, makes everything around it suffer. Other joints are forced to move differently. Muscles above and below alter their roles to compensate. Even the spine is impacted with the changes taking place around its 24 veterbral bones.

Three Steps to Prevent Injuries

Preventing injuries can encompass many factors involving your muscles, nutrition, footwear, weather, past medical history, mindset, warm-up, cool-down, equipment and so on. By now you know I like, no, I *love* to keep my sports medicine tips simple and positively impactful.

Keeping with my "simpler is better" approach, I've boiled my injury prevention down to three easy steps. Then I simply applied those three steps to your sport. Step 1 will help you identify overworked muscles needing treatment with your new self-myofascial unlocking skills, Step 2 shares sports medicine insight on which muscles need to be strengthened and, Step 3 recommends smart activities to prevent future injuries.

1. Unlock the motor muscles

With every sport, there are groups of muscles that do a large amount of the work. These prime movers are often referred to as the *agonist muscles*. That name sounds too stuffy for me. Instead, I call those blue-collar, hard-working muscles your *motor muscles*. They're your body's powerhouses to get the work done so you can enjoy your favorite sports and activities. Whichever muscle or muscle group comprises the motor muscles depends on the sport.

2. Strengthen opposing muscles

When the motor muscles are hard at work, opposing, or antagonistic, muscles are constantly being stretched and lengthened. These opposing muscles are located on the opposite side (front or back) of your body or limb. If the motor muscle is on the front side of an extremity, the opposing muscles are found on the back side of the limb. If the motor muscle is on the front side of the body, the opposing muscles are found on the back side of the body.

Opposing muscles are not recruited during specific sports to do most of the work, as the motor muscles are. Meanwhile, opposing muscles are consistently lengthened, thanks to the pull from motor muscles, so they tend to become overly long and weaker.

3. Launch prevention exercises for your sport

To avoid your body returning to an imbalanced and injury-prone state after a roller treatment, practice simple, preventative exercises designed to maintain your restored muscle balance.

Let's review the three-step plan: In Step 1, re-establish proper length of your motor muscles. In Step 2, identify opposing muscles which are too-long and too-weak and make them stronger. Here in Step 3, you're wisely launching a movement piggybacking on Steps 1 and 2 to prevent future injuries, keeping you in the game. In other words, to keep you in your "happy place."

Applying the Three Steps to Preventing Injuries in Your Sport

Here's where you apply the three steps to preventing injuries to your sport. Each sport has varying demands on your body. Each of the three steps is customized for your sport. Based on your sport below, you'll be instructed which muscle you need to unlock, which muscles need to be strengthened, and what movements/activities you should do to prevent injuries in the future.

REMEMBER

As always, listen to your muscles and joints. They will tell you what part of your daily routine you need to tweak or adjust. Your muscles and joints will thank you.

Running

Here's how to apply the three steps to prevent running-related injuries:

1. **Unlock the motor muscles.**

   - Hamstrings – Chapter 16

   - Hip flexors – Chapter 18

   - Chest — the pecs – Chapter 19

2. **Strengthen opposing muscles.**

   - Reverse lunges – Chapter 21

   - Bird dogs – Chapter 21

   - Prone reverse flies – Chapter 21

3. **Perform prevention exercises.**

   - Quad unlocking – Chapter 16

   - Lat and groin reach-out stretches – Chapter 21

   - Pool running

Cycling or spinning

Here's how to apply the three steps to prevent cycling- or spinning-related injuries:

1. **Unlock the motor muscles.**

   - Hip flexors – Chapter 18

   - Quads – Chapter 16

   - Chest — the pecs – Chapter 19

2. **Strengthen opposing muscles.**

   - Bird dogs – Chapter 21

   - Bridges – Chapter 21

   - Prone reverse flies – Chapter 21

3. **Perform prevention exercises.**

   - Hip flexor unlocking – Chapter 18

   - Aqua therapy/Swimming – Exercise in water is a great injury-preventing activity for athletes and non-athletes alike. Be it swimming, running in the deep end with a floatation device on, walking in the shallow end, or just moving your arms and legs against the resistance of the water, it's time well spent.

   - Lying face-up on a Swiss ball – Lying belly-up on a large (3 to 5 feet in diameter) Swiss ball is a heavenly position for a cyclist or anyone following prolonged sitting. If you think about it, laying face-up on a Swiss ball (lower spine extension) is the exact opposite position of a bicyclist (lower spine flexion). Lying belly-up on the Swiss ball lengthens your hip flexors, stretch your quads, and relax your abdominal muscles.

Gym weight training

Here's how to apply the three steps to prevent gym weight training-related injuries:

1. **Unlock the motor muscles.**

   - Chest — the pecs – Chapter 19

   - Biceps – Chapter 20

   - Lats – Chapter 19

2. **Strengthen opposing muscles.**

   - Rowing with bands – Chapter 21

   - Prone reverse flies – Chapter 21

   - Standing delt raises – Chapter 21

3. **Perform prevention exercises.**

   - Lat or groin reach-out stretches – Chapter 21

   - Resistive shoulder external rotation – Learn to master these exercises because they're key strength exercises for everyone who's active. With resistance originating from the opposite side of the body via a rubber exercise band, cable machine, or good old-fashioned manual resistance, forcefully externally rotate your lower arm outward with your elbow flexed to 90 degrees and inside of elbow held snuggly against your ribs directly below your armpit. Keep the motion slow in both directions and the resistance high enough for 8 to 12 reps per set for 3 to 5 sets.

   - Yoga/flexibility classes – Commit yourself to improving your posture with a flexibility expert. As a cyclist, your hip flexors and quads become strong, short and tight. Yoga classes or flexibility classes will help you "reverse ship" to make your hip flexors and quads strong, long and loose.

Swimming

Here's how to apply the three steps to prevent swimming-related injuries:

1. **Unlock the motor muscles.**

   - Chest — the pecs – Chapter 19

   - Lats – Chapter 19

   - Lower back extensors – Chapter 18

2. **Strengthen opposing muscles.**

   - Rowing with bands – Chapter 21

   - Prone reverse flies – Chapter 21

   - Crunches – Chapter 21

3. **Perform prevention exercises.**

   - Lat or groin reach-out stretches – Chapter 21

   - Chest or pecs stretches – Chapter 21

- Swimming the backstroke – Swimming the backstroke is a smart way to reverse your shoulder muscle firing patterns. The backstroke naturally adds balance to the muscles and fascia on the front/back of the chest/upper back as well as with your all-important rotator cuff.

Basketball

Here's how to apply the three steps to prevent basketball-related injuries:

1. Unlock the motor muscles.

- Quads – Chapter 16
- Calves – Chapter 17
- Groin – Chapter 16

2. Strengthen opposing muscles.

- Bridges – Chapter 21
- Wall sits, with toes off the ground – Chapter 21
- Side planks – Chapter 21

3. Perform prevention exercises.

- Lat or groin reach-out stretches – Chapter 21
- Pool running or swimming
- Bike riding – Bike riding is good for both your body and mind. It's easy on your joints with a reduction in compression, it can get you outside with the wind in your face, and it has a magical skill to make you feel half your age! Who can resist smiling and feeling less stressed when riding an outdoor bike? Not me and, hopefully, not you.

Golf

Here's how to apply the three steps to prevent golf-related injuries:

1. Unlock the motor muscles.

- Chest — the pecs – Chapter 19
- Abs – Chapter 18
- Hip flexors – Chapter 18

2. **Strengthen opposing muscles.**
   - Prone reverse flies – Chapter 21
   - Bird dogs – Chapter 21
   - Bridges – Chapter 21

3. **Perform prevention exercises.**
   - Chin tucks – Chapter 21
   - Lat or groin reach-out stretches – Chapter 21
   - Lying face-up on a Swiss ball

Soccer

Here's how to apply the three steps to prevent soccer-related injuries:

1. **Unlock the motor muscles.**
   - Quads – Chapter 16
   - Groin – Chapter 16
   - Calves – Chapter 17

2. **Strengthen opposing muscles.**
   - Bridges – Chapter 21
   - Side planks – Chapter 21
   - Wall sits, with toes off the ground

3. **Perform prevention exercises.**
   - Hip flexor stretches – Chapter 21
   - Calf stretches – Chapter 21
   - Bird dogs – Chapter 21

Tennis

Here's how to apply the three steps to prevent tennis-related injuries:

1. **Unlock the motor muscles.**
   - Lats – Chapter 19
   - Groin – Chapter 16
   - Quads – Chapter 16

2. **Strengthen opposing muscles.**

- Prone reverse flies – Chapter 21

- Side planks – Chapter 21

- Bridges – Chapter 21

3. **Perform prevention exercises.**

- Iliotibial band (ITB) stretches – Chapter 21

- Lat or groin reach-out stretches – Chapter 21

- Lying face-up on a Swiss ball

Gym cardio

Here's how to apply the three steps to prevent gym cardio-related injuries:

1. **Unlock the motor muscles.**

- Quads – Chapter 16

- Hip flexors – Chapter 18

- Calves – Chapter 17

2. **Strengthen opposing muscles.**

- Bird dogs – Chapter 21

- Bridges – Chapter 21

- Wall sits, with toes off the ground

3. **Perform prevention exercises.**

- Front planks – Chapter 21

- Hip flexor stretches – Chapter 21

- Groin stretches – Chapter 21

6

The Part of Tens

Learning what to *do* and what *not* to do with your rollers

Understanding the positive changes your body will make with your rollers

Identifying ten special groups who love their rollers

Chapter **24**
Ten Roller Do's and Don'ts

Full rollers, half rollers, handheld massagers, roller balls, and travel rollers have so many uses to keep you limber, pain-free, and active. You can use them at home, work, in your car, at the gym, inside and outdoors. They're easy to use and easy on your wallet. They give you a much better chance to stay in the game and out of the doctor's office.

But there are a few Do's and Don'ts to help you optimize the benefits of your rollers and keep you safe.

Do Breathe

Breathing allows your body to relax and your muscles to respond to the rollers. By breathing, you help your blood pressure and heart rate to stay low. A more relaxed body will benefit more from rolling and stretching. By holding your breath when your body is stressed by the roller, your blood pressure increases, your heart rate increases and your ability to relax the muscles being treated is lost.

Do Trust Your Roller and Your Body's Response

You will learn how the rollers feel and move while your body adapts to the pressure and motion of the rollers. Trust that relationship. Start slow, listen to your body, and use the pre-test/post-test program detailed in chapters 16–20 to determine how your muscles are responding to each treatment.

Do Be Creative

Once you've mastered my treatment programs in this book, be creative with your rollers and roller balls. Explore with different rollers, rolling patterns, and warmups to find what works best for you. Be creative while listening to your body to answer three simple questions:

>> What roller treatments help my muscles feel better?

>> What roller treatments increase my joint range of motions the most?

>> What roller treatments help my body to move better?

Do Toughen Up

Rollers can hurt. They can leave temporary marks and bruises, and cause discomfort. That's expected when you're unlocking muscles, fascia, and soft tissue that may have been cinched down for years. When you start to treat a new part of your body, you'll need to again put your game-face on and toughen up.

Do Follow Up Your Roll with Reset Moves

After each roll, educate your body on how to move with your extra-mobile muscles, fascia, and joints. Get off the roller to walk, dance, jump around, shadow box, or moon walk. Roll, then get up and move!

Don't Hold Your Breath

Breathing is so important I included it twice from two different angles. Just as I stated with my "Do Breathe" comment above, holding your breath defeats most of the benefits of rolling. Holding your breath is bad, period. Holding your breath is to your muscles similar to adding more air to a balloon. They both increase the internal pressure and make the outer "skin" tighter not looser.

Don't Roll on Swollen and Inflamed Injuries

Acute, or new, injuries with swelling and possibly bleeding won't benefit from a roller. With lots of healing to do after a new muscle tear or bruise, the pressure from a roller will probably accelerate the inflammation and prolong the healing time.

Don't Add Joint Motion Too Early

With my 56 roller treatments in Chapters 16 to 20, they include an easy-to-follow two-level treatment game plan. Level 1 uses static positions, and Level 2 includes dynamic movements to help you unlock your tight muscles faster.

WARNING

Adding Level 2 joint motion to a roller treatment should not be included until you and your muscles can handle it. The motion is a great way to unlock your muscles, but Level 2 is a progression you need to be properly prepared for.

Don't Work Against Your Body

Make your roller and your body allies on your journey to move better. Don't work *against* your body, work *with* your body.

Here's a healthy game plan:

1. **Roll.**
2. **Listen.**

3. **Test.**

4. **Adjust.**

5. **Re-roll.**

6. **Reassess.**

7. **Repeat.**

TIP

Read Chapter 8 for more details on this important topic.

Don't Roll on Nerves, Bones, or Open Wounds

Nerves, bones, and open wounds don't need a roller. In fact, rolling those three troubled tissues will increase your pain and delay your healing.

» **Understanding the physiological adaptation your body can make**

» **Planning for positive change with your quest to build a healthier body**

Chapter **25**

Ten Changes Your Body Will Feel from Rolling

As you become more flexible, more active, stronger, and healthier, your body will change. As you fight age, gravity, illness, and stress, your body will change. Change is inevitable in life. But you don't have to play a passive role as your body changes. Taking constructive actions can positively influence how your body changes. These positive active steps include a healthy diet, more exercise, drinking more water, getting more sleep, stretching more, regular medical exams, and the daily use of rollers.

Take a look at ten positive changes you will notice with your body when you add rollers to your daily wellness routine.

Looser Muscles

With less painful trigger points and more mobile myofascial tissue from using rollers, your muscles will have less tension applied to them. We've been programmed our whole lives to think if our muscles feel tight, they need to be stretched to release the knots. I can still hear my college track coach yelling at my middle-distance runner teammates and me: "Stretch, stretch, stretch!" Question: If you have a knot in your shoelaces, will stretching the knotted shoelace from both ends make it better or worse? Obviously stretching the shoelace will make the knot tighter and harder to release. Stretching a tight muscle will have the same effect.

Rolling allows a tight muscle and fascia to stretch and elongate sideways without adding tension to an already tight muscle. Rolling reduces the pressure being cinched down on the tight muscle by the surrounding fascia and the muscle itself. It's like taking duct tape off your muscles, allowing them to stretch in multiple directions as they were intended to do. See Chapter 8 to learn the priceless benefits of work with your muscles and not against your muscles.

Increased Joint Range of Motion

Muscles move joints. Therefore, when your muscles become looser following roller treatments, your joints will gain motion. The post-rolled muscles can move the joint through greater ranges because the muscles are now stronger. In addition, the rolled muscles stretch with less resistance when muscle on the opposite side of the joint are contracting.

Less Effort to Move

Looser muscles plus *More mobile joints* equals *Less energy needed to move those muscles and joints*. Using a roller frees restricted fascial tissue. This reduces the pressure being applied around the muscles, similar to taking off tight jeans before running five miles. It immediately reduces the effort needed to complete the five-mile run. To find out how to teach your body to move better with less effort, refer to Chapter 12.

Smellier Urine

This isn't a typo. Stream rolling your muscles with rollers will assist the muscles' ability to rid themselves of harmful toxins and waste products. Those waste products are the normal by-products of hard-working muscles. Thanks to the rollers, your lymphatic vessels become less restricted. The lymphatic system, an important waste-product drainage system for your extremities, can now easily drain the extra muscle-waste products into the bladder to be added to your urine.

As you will soon notice, the smell of your urine after using a roller will be stronger. That's kind of gross, I know, but it's a good thing to know.

Would you rather have those strong-smelling toxins in your muscles or in the toilet bowl?

Faster Warm-Up

I love to work out early in the morning. It's cooler here in Florida, the kids and dogs are still sleeping, and I can easily slip onto the plush golf courses to run without being cursed and run off the greens. But early rising means an early warm-up. (Ugh!) A 5:00 a.m. warm-up isn't too inviting. But the roller is the perfect early-morning warm-up partner for three reasons:

>> The roller hurts, so it wakes you up fast.

>> The roller is easy to use, so you don't have to think too much as your body and brain come to terms with the fact that you're no longer in your warm bed.

>> The roller is fast, so it reduces your warm-up time to mere minutes.

See Chapter 7 for elite warm-up tips.

Less Pain and Fewer Injuries

By helping your muscles to loosen up, your joints to increase their range, your body to move with less effort, your muscles to eliminate more of their waste products, and your warm-up to be more consistent, the roller helps you move and feel better. And with all those previously mentioned benefits, you'll have a reduced likelihood of pain and injury.

Tight muscles and compensations both during workouts and through your busy day are painful but, thanks to your rollers, they will be a thing of the past!

Increased Muscle Strength

When a muscle concentrically contracts, its muscle fibers shorten against a force while its opposing muscles lengthen. A muscle in pain and restriction cannot optimize its performance. Neither the muscle nor the brain will allow a strong muscle contraction if there is the threat of bodily harm. Envision what happens when you accidently step on a sharp object while walking barefoot. Your quad and calf muscle immediately turn off to reduce the pressure on your threatened foot.

Rollers eliminate painful muscle trigger points and relax tight muscle fascia. By doing so, your muscles are happier and stronger.

Improved Posture

When the troublemaker muscles — the pectoralis minor in the chest, the latissimus dorsi in the back and shoulder, and the hip flexors — are overly tight and strong, it results in poor posture. The solution is easy: unlock those muscles and strengthen their opposing muscles. See Chapter 9 for tips to improve your posture and Chapters 19 and 20 to discover how lengthen tight shoulder and upper back muscles. This is where you'll learn how to strengthen weak shoulder and upper back muscles for better posture in less than 10 minutes.

REMEMBER

Better muscle mobility, length, and strength on both sides of your body will translate into better posture.

Faster Recovery

After a hard workout or a hard day at work, your rollers will accelerate your recovery. Your muscles will be tired and stiff from the long day. Allowing the rollers to work their magic for five to ten minutes will help flush out the bad stuff (inflammation, lactic acid, and damaged blood cells), while allowing the good stuff (fresh blood and water) to easily enter the fatigued muscles. Mechanically, the roller steamrolls through the muscles, fascia, skin, fat, and all the fluid throughout the soft tissue. That alone will help your body to recover faster after a busy bout of work. See Chapter 9 for recovery techniques typically reserved for professional athletes.

Better Sleep

I've only taken one sleeping pill in my life; my sleeping secret is my roller. It's true, as my wife will confirm. I do two things every night before I put my head on my pillow, with an average fall asleep time of approximately two minutes:

1. **I roll my legs and hips.**

2. **I get on my knees to pray and express my gratitude.**

Think of all the physical benefits you will gain from rolling that are detailed throughout this book. Now imagine creating all those positive changes — like looser fascia, more relaxed muscles, and less waste products — in in your legs and hips. But then, immediately after you unlock you muscles, you just climb in bed and sleep.

TIP

Think about this for a minute. Instead of only using the roller to make those muscle and fascia changes before running down the road, lifting weights, or playing a hard game of tennis, now you'll able to use your new roller self-myofascial unlocking skills to relax your muscles and fascia to fall asleep faster and deeper!

The result: Your body is perfectly prepared for 8 hours of uninterrupted recovery time while you sleep like a baby. Give it a try.

Chapter **26**

Ten Groups Who Love Rollers

Rollers aren't for everyone, but for 80 percent of us, rollers rock! Let's take a look at ten groups of people who love rollers. Much like the happy man in Figure 26-1, these ten groups are different in many ways, but what they share is simple:

Rollers help them continue to _____.

What they put in the blank is up to them. It can be a popular sport like running or biking. It can be a strenuous workout like cross training or weightlifting. It can be a very personal activity like walking with a grandchild or recovering from a major surgery.

The "what" in the blank isn't important; it's personal, as it should be. The gratifying point here is that *rollers help people return to doing what they love to do.*

What will you put in the blank?

So, who are these ten groups who love rollers? Read on and find out!

Stiff or Inflexible People

If you're one of those individuals who always feels stiff and tight, you'll love rolling. Blame it on genetics, posture, age, or your lifestyle, but the fact is you may never have been overly flexible. A roller will plow through your tight muscles and fascia in minutes, giving you more flexibility than you may have gained following 30 minutes of boring stretching.

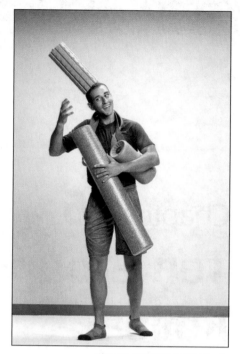

Photography by Haim Ariav & Klara Cu

FIGURE 26-1:
It's hard to hide this kind of love!

The Injury-Prone

The unfortunate people who always seem to be injured and in pain *need* to use a roller daily. Keeping muscles, tendons, fascia, and joints moving properly will reduce the risk of soft-tissue injury. By maintaining your flexibility and staying injury-free with your rollers and the details from this book, you'll achieve these three things:

>> You'll save yourself lots of *pain*.

>> You'll save yourself lots of *time*.

>> You'll save yourself lots of *money*.

Runners

By now you know how effective rollers are for keeping your muscles and fascia pliable, limber, and elastic. In other words, rollers keep your muscles "healthy." When it comes to the demanding sport of running, healthy muscles will keep you injury-free. Meanwhile, unhealthy muscles can easily lead to a painful injury.

Running is not kind to your leg muscles or joints. As the Law of Conservation of Energy taught us way back in our high school science classes, energy is neither created or destroyed. When we apply this law to our running, we now understand the force of our entire body slamming into the ground is being transferred into each of our legs as they strike the ground. The cushioning of our shoes absorbs some of that energy, but a large majority of the remaining force is immediately transferred to our legs.

As your foot slams into the ground, the massive forces are now racing up your leg. But thanks to your rolling and stretching routine, your quad and glute muscles are ready for the onslaught of high stress. Like a compressing spring, your quad and glute muscles effortlessly absorb the loads with smooth lengthening (eccentric) contractions. Your now-loaded muscles are just waiting to release their new energy when the compressed leg is allowed to push off the ground.

In contrast, a rigid, un-rolled, and therefore unhealthy leg muscles aren't prepared for the rapidly approaching high forces racing up the leg. So what do they do? They selfishly only think of protecting themselves. The weak, tight leg muscles lock down with a strong isometric (static, no motion) contraction. In doing so, per the Law of Conservation of Energy, every pound of the remaining energy is now transferred into your joints, mostly your knees and hips, with pain and injury not far behind.

REMEMBER

When healthy, loose and stretchy muscles are loaded when running, they absorb the forces like a giant spring. When unhealthy, tight and rigid muscles are loaded when running, they absorb the forces like a brick.

Take-home point: If you're a runner, you need to be a roller.

Mature Athletes

While I recently stretched on a beach with my 11-year old son, I leaned to my side, spanning one hand skyward with the other desperately reaching for the sand, but stopping well short of my optimistic goal. Meanwhile, my son mirrored my stretch, with his 11-year-old spine effortlessly bent sideways, with his hand buried deep in the sand. "That's *sad*, Dad, so sad," he said empathetically.

For those of us north of 40 years old (the "mature athletes," as I like to call us), our muscles seem to stretch more like leather belts, compared to youthful and stretchy muscles, which stretch like rubber bands. Mature athletes desperately need the assistance of rollers to maintain less fascial restrictions on their tighter muscles and joints.

Cross Trainers

Cross training involves a variety of exercises such as cardio conditioning, strength training, agility drills, balance training, core strengthening, climbing, ballistic drills, carrying exercises, and plyometric routines. In other words, cross trainers' bodies work hard to do a lot of different types of intense workouts. Their entire muscular system is constantly overloaded, and their muscles are consistently in need of recovery. The use of rollers before a workout, as part of the workout, and following the workout is the routine for smart cross trainers to keep them injury-free in a very demanding sport.

Bikers

Bikers put a high demand on their quads and hip flexors in a restricted position on the bike, as shown in Figure 26-2. Unlocking their quads, hip flexors, and lower back before and after a ride using a roller or roller ball will improve performance and prevent injury.

FIGURE 26-2: A prolonged compressed hip posture on a bike increases the need for a roller both before and after you get on the saddle.

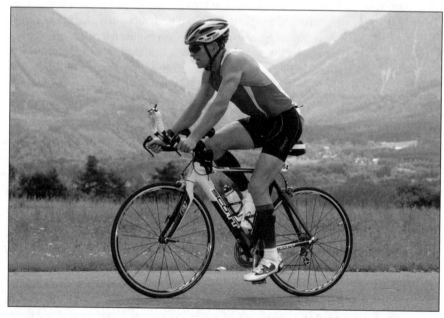

Photography by Haim Ariav & Klara Cu

Stop-and-Go Athletes

Athletes who do a lot of change of directions during their sport, like tennis, basketball, volleyball, and frisbee, put high stress on their tendons and muscles. These are the types of athletes who often suffer from tendonitis, an inflammation of the tendon, because of the rapid loads placed on their tendons and muscles during their sport.

The more pliable, flexible, and responsive their muscles are, the better prepared the tendons are to remain injury-free during stop-and-go sports. With tendons positioned on both ends of a muscle to anchor the muscle to the bones, much of the health of the tendon is reliant on the health of its muscles. Healthy and responsive muscles handle high forces with ease, which in turn protects the tendons.

Think about anyone you know who has ruptured or torn an Achilles tendon, patella tendon, hamstring, calf, groin, or quad muscle. They were probably doing some type of ballistic, quick, change of direction type movement.

Walkers and Hikers

If you think walking isn't a difficult task for the body, think again. Walking may not apply a lot of stress to your muscles, tendons, and joints, but its high volume within a small range of motion makes it difficult for lower-extremity muscles to stay flexible. You take approximately 2000 steps per mile when you walk, with all of those steps in a short, confined range of motion. Rollers help a walker or hiker's tight muscles and fascia to stay looser, reduce trigger points, increase blood flow, and recover faster.

The ability to travel with a roller and use it in the gym, in the park, or at the top of a mountain makes rollers a perfect training partner for hikers, walkers, trail runners, hunters, and even bird watchers.

Human Cardio Machines

When I watch the impressive "human cardio machines" in the gym jump from one cardio machine to the next, I'm in awe of their stamina and focus. They seem like massive lungs with legs as they sweat on the treadmill before switching to the spin bike, then the elliptical, and then the rower. I love their cross-training routines as they wisely enhance their endurance and strength. The diverse loads on their muscles desperately need the assistance of a roller to stay limber.

Yoga Haters

"I hate yoga," is a phrase I hear on a weekly basis. And a note to the yogis out there: Don't shoot the messenger! I'm just quoting the yoga haters.

Personally, I like yoga. But not everyone shares my opinion. For those who despise stretching and find stretching classes both boring and ineffective, rolling is the perfect substitute. The roller treatments in chapters 16 to 20 and the roller workouts/stretches in Chapter 21 *will* get you limber and strong faster than you ever imagined. Rolling is quick, effective, and it's not yoga.

Index

I

iliacus muscle, 240

iliotibial band. *See* ITB

impingement syndrome, 350–351

infection, fascia and, 153

inflammation

  fascia and, 153

  inflammation phase of scar healing, 159

  rolling and, 385

injury management

  ankle

    Achilles tendonitis, 369–370

    arthritis, 368–369

  elbow

    golfer's elbow, 354–355

    tennis elbow, 353–354

  hip

    hip flexor strain, 359–360

    hip rotator strain, 360–361

    overview, 358

  injury prone people, 394

  knee

    chondromalacia, 366–367

    patella tendonitis, 365–366

  lower back

    glute pain, 357–358

    overview, 355–356

    pain, 357

  overview, 15–16, 345–346

  ROLLER Treatment Planner

    execute treatment plan, 350

    lay out treatment plan, 349

    listening to body, 347

    origin of restrictions, 347

    overview, 16, 346–347

    research, 347

    reset moves, 350

  shoulder

    impingement syndrome, 350–351

    rotator cuff strain, 351–352

  thigh

    hamstring strain, 363–364

    overview, 361–362

    quadriceps strain, 362–363

injury prevention

  avoiding injury when rolling, 61–63

  basketball, 378

  cardio training, 380

  cycling or spinning, 376

  golf, 378–379

  overview, 17, 371–373

  post-workout recovery, 107

  prevention exercises, 374–375

  running, 375

  soccer, 379

  strengthening opposing muscles, 374

  swimming, 377–378

  tennis, 379–380

  unlocking motor muscles, 374

  weight training, 376–377

integumentary system, 140

isometric muscle contraction, 115

ITB (iliotibial band)

  overview, 194–195, 198–199

  preparing for rolling, 195, 199

  stretching, 341

  unlocking, 195–198, 199–203

J

James, LeBron, 140

joints

  arthritis, 116

  bones and, 115–116

  joint injury pain, 180

  muscles and

    cardiovascular system, 140

    coordinating, 141–142

    digestive system, 140

    endocrine system, 140

    general discussion, 139–142

    Golgi tendon organs, 143

    integumentary system, 140

    lymphatic system, 140

    muscular system, 140

    nervous system, 140

    orthopedic compensations, 146–150

    reproductive system, 140

posture and, 148–149

scar tissue and, 148

temporary pain and, 147

outdoor settings, 42

P

padding and pressure relief, 33, 43–44

pain

associated with scar tissue, 161–162

bone injury, 180–181

finding sources of, 179–182

good pain vs. bad pain, 60, 99–101

joint injury, 180

management vs. avoidance, 76

mindset toward, 82–83

muscle injury, 179–180

nerve injury, 181

related to orthopedic compensations, 147–148

as sign of overaggressive rolling, 78

sources of muscle pain, 121

tight fascia, 181–182

"painful grapes." *See* trigger points

patella tendonitis, 365–366

pectoral muscles (pecs)

overview, 261–262

preparing for rolling, 262–263

unlocking, 263–265

pelvis, 130–131

peroneal muscles

overview, 218

preparing for rolling, 219

unlocking, 219–222

physiological changes, due to warming up, 83–84

Physio-pedia.com, 117

plantar flexion, 210

positive thinking, 82

posterior forearm

overview, 297–298

preparing for rolling, 298–299

unlocking, 299–301

posture, 13

avoiding injuries, 63

effects of rolling on, 390

evaluating

feet, 131–132

head, 127–128

lower back, 129–130

pelvis, 130–131

shoulders, 128–129

fascia and, 153

forward head, 258

importance of, 123–125

overview, 125–126

rounded shoulders, 258

sitting, 133–134

squatting, 177–178

standing, 133, 171–173

symptoms of poor posture

lower back, 135

neck and upper back, 134

shoulders, 135

tips for improving, 135–137

walking, 174–176

post-workout recovery

mistakes to avoid, 109

overview, 103

Six-Minute Recovery Roll-Down, 104–107

stretching, 108–109

value of, 104

preventative medicine. *See also* injury prevention

post-workout recovery, 107

roller treatments as, 17

proliferation phase, scar healing, 159

psoas major muscle, 240

psoas minor muscle, 240

PVC piping, 49

Q

quadriceps (quads)

overview, 189–190

preparing for rolling, 190

quadriceps strain, 362–363

stretching, 340

unlocking, 190–194

Quigley, Colleen, 56

R

reciprocal inhibition, 95–96
rectus femoris muscle (upper quad), 240
relaxing environment, 39, 42
remodeling phase, scar healing, 159
repetitive motion, fascia and, 153
reproductive system, 140
reset moves, 384
resistance bands, 34
respiratory system, 140
restrictive adhesions, fascia and, 153
reverse lunges, 334–335
roller balls, 26–27. *See also* rollers
ROLLER Treatment Planner, 16
  execute treatment plan, 350
  lay out treatment plan, 349
  listening to body, 347
  origin of restrictions, 347
  overview, 346–347
  research, 347
  resetting way of moving, 350
roller treatments. *See* injury management; injury prevention
roller workouts
  core and spine
    strengthening exercises, 321–328
    stretches, 329–331
  lower-body
    overview, 331
    strengthening exercises, 332–339
    stretches, 339–342
  overview, 14–15, 305–306
  strengthening, 306–307
  stretching, 307–308
  upper-body
    overview, 308–309
    strengthening exercises, 309–318
    stretches, 319–320
rollers
  accessories
    chair and balance dowel, 32
    handheld massager, 30–31
    handheld rollers, 30–31

    padding and pressure relief, 33
    resistance bands, 34
    stretch bands, 34
    yoga mat, 31
  cylindrical rollers, 9, 21–22
  half rollers, 9, 27
  multi-pattern rollers, 22–23
  overview, 20–21
  roller balls, 9, 26–27
  selecting, 8–9, 35
  travel rollers, 28
  types of, 20–28
  vibrating rollers, 23–25
rolling. *See also* self-myofascial unlocking
  best times to roll, 69–72
  effects of
    faster recovery, 390
    faster warm-up, 389
    improved posture, 390
    improved sleep, 391
    increased muscles strength, 389–390
    increased range of motion, 388
    looser muscles, 387–388
    reduced pain and injury, 389
    smelly urine, 388–389
  having sufficient space, 40
  improvising, 38–41
  outdoors, 42
  overview, 37
  padding and pressure relief, 43–44
  pre-bedtime rolling, 72–75
  relaxing environment, 39, 42
  when not to roll, 75–78
  when traveling, 57
"roof" muscles (glutes), 12–13
  overview, 249–251
  preparing for rolling, 252
  unlocking, 252–255
rotator cuff strain, 351–352
rubber rollers, 49
running/runners, 375, 394–395

About the Author

Mike D. Ryan, PT, ATC, CES, PES, is a sports medicine specialist, physical therapist, and former National Football League (NFL) head athletic trainer with the Jacksonville Jaguars and New York Giants. A sports medicine analyst for *NBC Sports* and *Sunday Night Football,* Mike has focused his post-NFL career on teaching individuals, young and old, the art of restoring pain-free joint movement without medicine.

Mike continues to expand his role as a leader in sports medicine, as both a sports injury management expert and an elite endurance athlete. He has completed six Ironman triathlons in five countries (posting his personal best time of 10 hours and 36 minutes at the age of 46), represented Team USA in the 2002 Duathlon World Championships, and completed the Ironman World Championship in 1994.

Presently in his late 50s, Mike continues to compete in Spartan Races, road-running races, and challenging endurance events throughout the U.S. each year. Mike is also an extreme-sport enthusiast whose unique accomplishments include acrobatic plane wing–walking, Running of the Bulls in Spain, great white shark diving in South Africa, boogie boarding on the Zambezi River in Zimbabwe, three Escape from Alcatraz Triathlons, three Empire State Building Run-Up races in NYC, and cave rafting in Belize.

As the founder of Mike Ryan Sports Medicine, Inc., Mike is a popular consultant to professional athletes, corporate athletes, and sports medicine specialists across the country, reinforcing his simple mission statement: To enhance the health of others.

During his 26 years in the NFL, Mike served as President of the Professional Football Athletic Trainers Society Research and Education Foundation from 1999 to 2014; Chairman of the NFL Collegiate Athletic Trainers Committee; a member of the Professional Football Athletic Trainers Society's Executive Committee; and a member of the NFL Foot and Ankle Committee.

He is proud of his role as a mentor for young sports medicine professionals. Three of his former NFL assistants have been employed as head athletic trainers in the NFL: Andre Tucker with the Chicago Bears, Joe Sheehan with the Cleveland Browns, and John Burrell with the Washington Football Team.

Mike attended Central Connecticut State University, earning his degree in athletic training before earning his physical therapy degree from the University of Connecticut.

Dedication

To painful trigger points and overly tight fascia,
You've haunted my friends for way too long.
Your reign is over!

United with rollers,
Mike

Author's Acknowledgments

Dept. of Loving Support: Samantha Ryan, Gannon Ryan, Makayla Ryan, Penny (dog), and Teddy (dog)

Editorial Support: Tracy Boggier, Chrissy Guthrie, Kristie Pyles, Marylouise Wiack

Photography and Graphics: Haim Ariav, Klara Cu, Jonathan DelRosario, Rick Wilson

Author Mentors: Jon Gordon, Barbara Pinson-Lash

Photo Studio Host: Richard Cooper

Models: Russ Allen, Haim Ariav, Sara Ariav, Caleb Cooper, Klara Cu, Crystal Davis, Chris Gambino, Sarah Hernandez, Bruce Jackson, Maurice Jones-Drew, Noel Medina, Asjah Muhammad, Montell Owens, Lisa Owens, Colleen Quigley, Joe Rivera, Marielle Rodriguez-Mundy, Gannon Ryan, Makayla Ryan, Samantha Ryan, Brett Simpson, Bec Wilcox, Joleen Young, Michael Young, Thomas Young

Publisher's Acknowledgments

Senior Acquisitions Editor: Tracy Boggier

Managing Editor: Kristie Pyles

Editorial Project Manager and Development Editor: Christina N. Guthrie

Copy Editor: Marylouise Wiack

Production Editor: Mohammed Zafar Ali

Photographers: Haim Ariav, Klara Cu

Cover Image: Haim Ariav

Take dummies with you everywhere you go!

Whether you are excited about e-books, want more from the web, must have your mobile apps, or are swept up in social media, dummies makes everything easier.

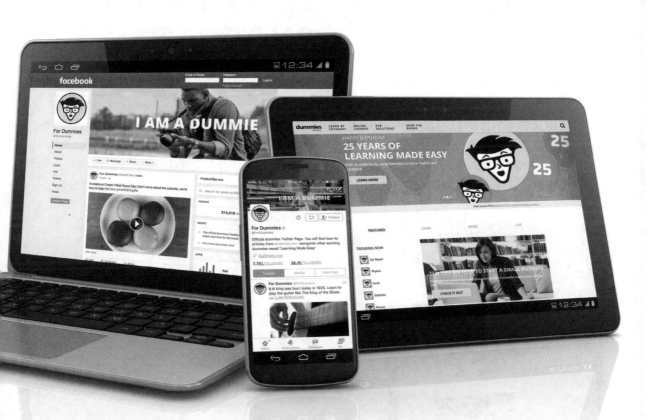

Find us online!

     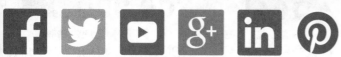

dummies.com

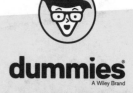

dummies®
A Wiley Brand

Dummies is the global leader in the reference category and one of the most trusted and highly regarded brands in the world. No longer just focused on books, customers now have access to the dummies content they need in the format they want. Together we'll craft a solution that engages your customers, stands out from the competition, and helps you meet your goals.

Advertising & Sponsorships

Connect with an engaged audience on a powerful multimedia site, and position your message alongside expert how-to content. Dummies.com is a one-stop shop for free, online information and know-how curated by a team of experts.

- Targeted ads
- Video
- Email Marketing
- Microsites
- Sweepstakes sponsorship

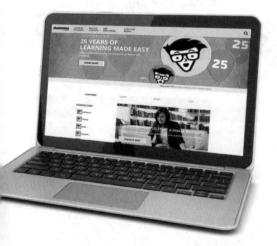

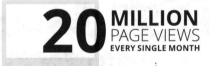

20 MILLION PAGE VIEWS
EVERY SINGLE MONTH

15 MILLION UNIQUE
VISITORS PER MONTH

43%
OF ALL VISITORS
ACCESS THE SITE
VIA THEIR MOBILE DEVICES

700,000 NEWSLETTER SUBSCRIPTION
TO THE INBOXES OF
300,000 UNIQUE INDIVIDUALS **EVERY WEEK**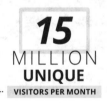

# of dummies

Custom Publishing

Reach a global audience in any language by creating a solution that will differentiate you from competitors, amplify your message, and encourage customers to make a buying decision.

- Apps
- Books
- eBooks
- Video
- Audio
- Webinars

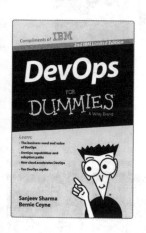
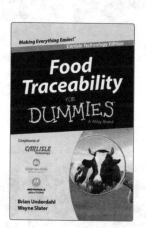
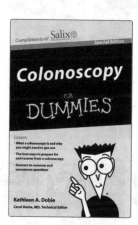
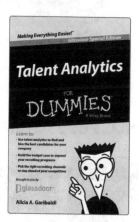

Brand Licensing & Content

Leverage the strength of the world's most popular reference brand to reach new audiences and channels of distribution.

For more information, visit **dummies.com/biz**

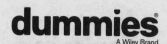

PERSONAL ENRICHMENT

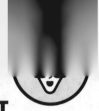
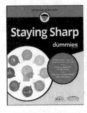 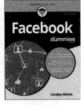 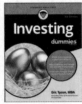 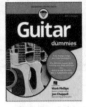 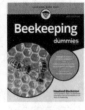 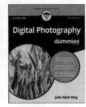
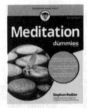 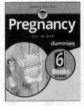 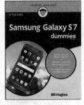 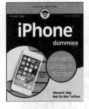 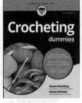 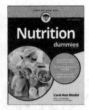
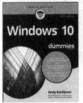 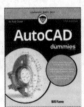 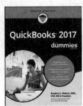 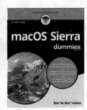 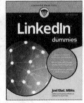 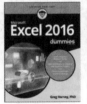 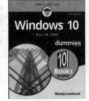
  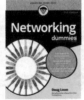 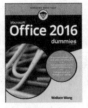 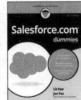